HIV/AIDS
IN SPORT

HIV/AIDS IN SPORT

IMPACT, ISSUES, AND CHALLENGES

Gopal Sankaran, MD, Dr.PH
Karin A. E. Volkwein, PhD
Dale R. Bonsall, M.Ed

West Chester University of Pennsylvania

Editors

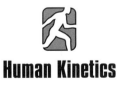

Human Kinetics

Library of Congress Cataloging-in-Publication Data

HIV/AIDS in sport : impact, issues, and challenges / Gopal Sankaran,
Karin A. E. Volkwein, Dale R. Bonsall.
     p.   cm.
Includes bibliographical references and index.
ISBN 0-88011-749-4
  1. AIDS (Disease)   2. Sport medicine.   3. Athletes--Diseases.
4. Athletes--Health and hygiene.   I. Sankaran, Gopal, 1954-   .
II. Volkwein, Karin A. E., 1959-   .   III. Bonsall, Dale R., 1938-   .
RA644.A25H575523   1999
362.1'969792'0088796--dc21   98-37052
                                                        CIP

ISBN: 0-88011-749-4

Acquisitions Editor: Loarn Robertson; **Developmental Editor:** Kristine Enderle;
Assistant Editor: Amy Flaig; **Copyeditor:** Michelle Sandifer; **Proofreader:** Jim Burns;
Indexer: Sharon Duffy; **Graphic Designer:** Keith Blomberg; **Graphic Artist:** Denise
Lowry; **Cover Designer:** Jack Davis; **Printer:** Versa Press

Printed in the United States of America   10   9   8   7   6   5   4   3   2   1

Human Kinetics
Web site: http://www.humankinetics.com/

United States: Human Kinetics, P.O. Box 5076, Champaign, IL 61825-5076
1-800-747-4457
e-mail: humank@hkusa.com

Canada: Human Kinetics, 475 Devonshire Road Unit 100, Windsor, ON N8Y 2L5
1-800-465-7301 (in Canada only)
e-mail: humank@hkcanada.com

Europe: Human Kinetics, P.O. Box IW14, Leeds LS16 6TR, United Kingdom
(44) 1132 781708
e-mail: humank@hkeurope.com

Australia: Human Kinetics, 57A Price Avenue, Lower Mitcham, South Australia 5062
(088) 277 1555
e-mail: humank@hkaustralia.com

New Zealand: Human Kinetics, P.O. Box 105-231, Auckland 1
(09) 523 3462
e-mail: humank@hknewz.com

Dedicated to the memory of
David Schultz
(June 6, 1959 – January 26, 1996)
an international wrestler,
who planted the seed for this book.

It is our hope that
the Human Immunodeficiency Virus
will be eradicated
in the near future.

AIDS Memorial Sculpture

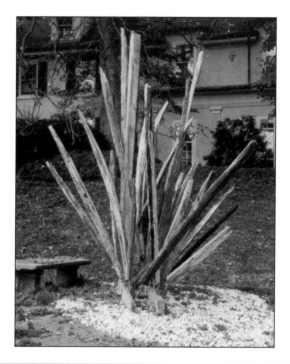

AIDS Memorial Sculpture for Gay Men's Health Crisis, New York, New York, November 1997; Sculpted by James A. Caplan, Bryn Mawr, Pennsylvania.

Todestanz

Some die alone
Some die embraced
Time suffers endless thoughts
This slow Dance of Death

Contents

Foreword

Jack Harvey
Chief Physician of USA Wrestling

The physical nature of wrestling carries with it the risk of injury. Fortunately, most of the injuries that occur are minor. They include lacerations and nosebleeds that are often managed on the mat during injury time-out. A decade ago, injury time-out often was not even required for minor instances of bleeding. More serious problems were quickly taped, and the injured combatants allowed to continue the match soon. Today, the threat of blood-borne infectious agents such as hepatitis B and human immunodeficiency virus (HIV) have markedly changed how blood is dealt with during training and competition. Universal precautions such as the use of rubber gloves, decontamination solutions, and special containers are evident during wound care. Rule changes have evolved over the past few years. They now mandate immediate stoppage of a bout in which the referee sees any bleeding. In many cases, additional injury time-out is allowed to close and clean wounds adequately as well as clean blood from uniforms and mats.

Despite these advances, the threat of serious infections still looms over sport and especially over contact sports such as wrestling. Research and education about the care of the bleeding wrestler has to continue and expand. Rule changes still need to be forthcoming, especially in international wrestling. The rules currently permit one or more time-outs for the "accidentally" untied shoelace or the obvious feigned injury needed by an exhausted wrestler. However, the regulations limit blood time-outs to two minutes rather than a more reasonable five minutes as occurs in high school or the National Collegiate Athletic Association (NCAA). Have policy makers forgotten that stopping bleeding, covering the wound, and removing blood from the playing surface actually protect the noninjured opponent? These procedures do not merely save him or her from a minor skin infection that can be controlled or cured with creams or oral medications but from a disease without a cure that has an 85% fatality rate. Also remember that HIV is a sport injury that affects not only the athlete but can infect and kill his or her spouse or partner.

Recently, the author surveyed the team members of a Pan-American team to determine their level of concern about blood-borne pathogens and how the National Governing Body (NGB) was dealing with the problem. Twenty-four wrestlers out of 26 returned the questionnaires. The Greco-Roman team returned nine forms, men's freestyle returned nine forms, and women's freestyle returned six forms. Sixty percent of the men were quite concerned with the risk of blood-borne pathogens in wrestling, and 50% supported mandatory testing of participants. Sixty percent of the male wrestlers expressed concerns about the risk for spouses or significant others. Interestingly, 100% of the female respondents were not worried at all about these risks in wrestling, either for themselves or for their spouses. Over 90% of all respondents felt that officials and trainers were doing a good job of dealing with the blood exposures on the mat.

While it is gratifying that the majority of the athletes in this survey feel that the medical staff and officials in international wrestling are doing a good job dealing with the blood-borne pathogen problem, some areas of concern remain. The rules for blood time-out need to be liberalized from the Fédération Internationale des Luttes Associées (FILA), increasing them from two minutes to a more reasonable five minutes. Athletes raise the question of mandatory testing. The NGB and FILA need to address this issue despite the legal problems surrounding such testing. Finally, lack of concern by the interviewed athletes may suggest that such a cavalier attitude stems from inadequate education of the teams rather than a blind faith in the efficacy of the medical team. More work needs to be done in athlete education for both males and females because this problem is not going to go away. This book is a step in the right direction to educate all those involved in sport.

Introduction to HIV/AIDS in Sport

Gopal Sankaran, Karin A. E. Volkwein, and Dale R. Bonsall
West Chester University of Pennsylvania

People around the world have arrived at a crossroad in the history of the acquired immunodeficiency syndrome (AIDS) epidemic. The death toll continues to rise and the faces of those infected continue to change. In the United States alone, an estimated 650,000–900,000 people are infected with the human immunodeficiency virus (HIV). AIDS is the most serious disease to appear in modern times. As of this writing, neither a vaccine nor a cure is in sight. Therefore, the disease, once acquired, will ultimately lead to death. Although most scientific experts agree that HIV is the basic cause of AIDS, social factors—mainly lifestyle—significantly affect the extent to which the virus is transmitted. In the past, it was believed that AIDS was concentrated among homosexuals (gays) and injecting drug users (IDUs). To date, the fastest-growing groups of people acquiring HIV in the United States are women and children. Hence, no one is excluded from contracting HIV if proper precautions are *not* followed.

In recent years, the media has focused on professional athletes who have tested HIV-positive. This raises the question of whether HIV can be acquired through interactions while playing sport. The National Collegiate Athletic Association (NCAA) has estimated that 0.08% of athletes are HIV positive compared with 0.02% of nonathletes (Kersey 1994). The American Medical Society for Sports Medicine and the American Academy of Sport Medicine recognize that HIV poses a series of important and complex issues for practitioners involved in the care of athletes. Speculation and misconceptions have occurred regarding the possibility of HIV transmission through sport. Based on limited information and irrational fear, athletes have been excluded from sporting competitions or have been encouraged to retire prematurely from their sporting careers. In other cases, athletes have been subjected to random HIV testing prior to sporting encounters. Are these practices justified? What proper procedures should be followed? Where do sporting professionals, such as athletic trainers, turn for information?

HIV/AIDS in Sport provides an overview of HIV infection, the resultant AIDS, and their impact on sport. The book draws upon the knowledge of experts from multiple disciplines, including health, kinesiology, sports medicine, law, sociology, psychology, and philosophy. This volume is written to answer questions raised by health professionals, physical education professionals, preservice health and physical education students, athletes (both amateurs and professionals), and sport personnel (such as athletic trainers and administrators, sports medicine specialists, coaches, teachers, fitness trainers, and exercise physiologists). The book addresses guidelines for testing, making ethical decisions, and dealing with social, psychological, and legal issues. It also discusses strategies to prevent and control the spread of HIV.

The text examines common myths and misconceptions about HIV transmission and AIDS (chapter 1), followed by an accurate account of medical facts about HIV disease (chapter 2). The book also analyzes the impact of HIV in sport, including the effects of exercise on the immune system and on AIDS (chapter 3). Furthermore, the role of the game official in prevention and taking measures to control HIV infection in sport is discussed (chapter 4). The text also addresses the psychological and social ramifications that athletes face when they are found to be HIV positive, including a discussion of the effect of HIV infection on professional and amateur athletes' daily lives both on and off the field (chapters 5 and 6). Ethical aspects (chapters 7 and 8) and legal issues (chapter 9) pertaining to HIV in sport are the final subjects discussed in this text. The book also discusses problems related to whether the HIV-infected athlete should be allowed to participate in sport, and a review of current legislation and judicial findings is provided (conclusion).

Ethical questions are complex in nature. No simple right or wrong answers exist, and the process by which an ethical decision can be derived is rather complicated. In order to avoid a one-sided perspective, we have chosen to include two chapters about HIV and ethics in this book. Chapter 7 discusses the issue using examples from the perspective of the athletes, while chapter 8 investigates the issue from the perspective of the sport practitioner, specifically the athletic trainer. The authors hope that both perspectives, along with the rationalization for an ethical framework, will provide the readers with the basic tools to derive their own ethical conclusions regarding HIV and sport.

A glossary of terms and a guide to resources for HIV/AIDS are included for the reader's reference. The resources section includes phone numbers and addresses of national organizations, phone numbers for state hot lines for HIV/AIDS information, as well as websites for some of the leading professional journals and organizations. Readers are encouraged to consult them for additional information.

This book is intended to serve as a guideline in five ways. First, it will help readers understand HIV and AIDS as they relate to sport. Second, it will help them comprehend the magnitude of HIV infection in the United States and the modes of transmission. Third, this book will promote understanding of the disease and the individuals affected by it. Fourth, it will help professionals develop ethical and moral reasoning for policy implementation related to HIV-positive athletes in their institutions. Fifth, this book will help sports medicine personnel devise practical preventive and control measures. Education remains the key in the effort to prevent blood-borne pathogen transmission. Sports medicine personnel play an important role in educating athletes, their families, athletic trainers, health care providers, coaches, and officials involved in sport.

References

Kersey, R.D. (1994). *Anabolic-Androgenic Steroid Use Among California Community College Student-Athletes.* Unpublished doctoral dissertation, University of New Mexico. Cited in Bryant, J., & McElroy, M. (1997). *Sociological Dynamics of Sport and Exercise.* Englewood, CO: Morton.

CHAPTER 1

Transmission of HIV in Sport

Karin A. E. Volkwein and Dale R. Bonsall
West Chester University of Pennsylvania

The announcement made on November 7, 1991, that the famous basketball star Earvin "Magic" Johnson had tested positive for antibodies to the human immuno-deficiency virus (HIV), left the world wondering whether HIV can be transmitted through professional and amateur sports, especially contact sports. Every tabloid ran headlines and every locker room had rumors concerning possible transmission of HIV during a contest. Blood spills are common during a sporting contest, especially in contact sports. Thus, people interpreted Magic's subsequent voluntary retirement from the Los Angeles Lakers as the most sensible reaction at that time. Most called this decision heroic and ethical. At that time, the general population believed that a person with HIV/AIDS had the responsibility to do nothing that would jeopardize coworkers, place team members at risk, or create anxieties. Thus, most people expected a person with the deadly virus to retire or take a leave of absence. Thereafter, Magic was reinstated and continued to play basketball for the Lakers. He has since retired. Has the threat of HIV transmission through sport been eliminated? Is the risk real or imagined?

In the meantime, professional boxer Tommy Morrison tested positive in 1996 for HIV. Due to society's pressure, his first reaction was to retire from the sport of boxing. This seemed to be the most logical conclusion since other states followed in the footsteps of the Nevada Boxing Association's 1988 mandate to ban HIV-positive athletes from participating in boxing contests. Later, Morrison returned to the boxing ring for one last glorious fight on behalf of those who, like himself, are infected with HIV. Although the national Centers for Disease Control and Prevention have received no reports of HIV transmission through sport, various other state amateur and professional sports organizations continue to enforce rules to prevent HIV-infected athletes from competing in sporting competitions. This includes all contact and some noncontact sports (McGrew et al. 1993).

Are any of these bans on HIV-positive sport professionals justified? What do we do with athletes who wish to continue to pursue their athletic careers after testing HIV positive? HIV-positive athletes do exist and compete in professional and intercollegiate sports. The exact number of such athletes is difficult to obtain. Then, what is the actual risk of HIV transmission in various sports?

Determining the actual risk of HIV transmission in different sports is difficult. A scientific risk analysis would have to take into account the following parameters: the number of people the athlete may come into close contact with, the percentage of those people who are HIV-infected, the frequency of possible intense-contact situations in a given sport, and the risk of infection per possible contact. Even if one could possibly devise a statistically correct percentage concerning the risk for HIV transmission in a given sport, this percentage would be extremely small. However, it would *not* be zero. Thus, the question remains for every sport professional, what is an acceptable risk?

Participation in sport is never risk free; in fact, no situation in life comes without risk. However, people generally try to minimize risks as much as possible, for instance, by wearing a seat belt while driving a car or a helmet when mountain biking. However, it is impossible to rule out every risk. That is a fact of life. Nevertheless, it is prudent to determine the situations where HIV is most likely to be transmitted. This chapter discusses the relative risks of allowing HIV-infected athletes to compete in all levels of sporting competition.

Attitudes Toward HIV-Positive People

Objectively assessing the actual risk of HIV infection rather than letting emotions or fear dictate philosophy and policy is vital. To date, the public continues to have many misconceptions about HIV and AIDS. Consequently, HIV-positive individuals suffer from discrimination and elimination from jobs and from sport. They are being ostracized by "friends."

> "We have no right to point fingers" in the U.S. . . . citing calls for mandatory testing and segregation . . . people's attitudes toward those with AIDS are closely linked with their attitudes toward minorities, especially gays. "The same variables that predict prejudice toward homosexuals, blacks and religious minorities can be used to predict attitudes toward" people with AIDS. (United Press International 1989).

The knowledge disseminated about HIV and AIDS has dramatically changed over the past 15 years. However, has the perception among the general public changed as well? When the developed world was first informed about HIV at the beginning of the 1980s, people often referred to the disease as the demise of gays and drug users. Today we know that no one is excluded from contracting HIV if that person does not take proper precautions. Currently, the fastest-growing infected groups of people are women and children. HIV spreads across gender lines, ethnic and racial backgrounds, as well as social class and age categories.

A study conducted in 1991 found that college students' perception about those with AIDS is linked to their attitudes toward homosexuality. This study determined that most students are accepting of people with AIDS, but tolerance can differ. Females tolerate people with AIDS more than males do. Even though most students are accepting, they tolerate individuals who contracted the disease through a blood transfusion more than those who contracted it through a sexual encounter. Students are more likely to evade social contact with the latter group of HIV-infected individuals. Students tolerate heterosexuals with AIDS more than homosexuals with AIDS. The results of the study indicated antigay prejudice and the perception of AIDS as primarily a gay problem (United Press International 1991).

The findings of the study are significant, and perhaps they still reflect the attitudes most people hold today toward people with AIDS. Attitudes are hard to change but can be influenced through education. However, the interviewed students reflected views of people who formed their perceptions at an educational institution. By now, the students have probably carried these attitudes with them into the workforce. Thus, attitudes toward HIV-infected individuals have probably not changed drastically during the last seven years since the study was conducted. These attitudes about HIV-infected people are based on emotions rather than on objective reasoning.

Despite a historic drop in AIDS cases and deaths in the United States during the last few years, the rate at which people become infected with HIV has held relatively steady. The attitude of some people infected with HIV seems to reflect carelessness. For example, Tommy Morrison seems to disregard HIV as a serious disease, and medical experts are concerned that he might be promoting carelessness with regard to health care and lifestyle. Morrison was quoted as having said that he does not take prescribed medications and that the infection "doesn't seem like that big of a deal" (USA Today 1996). However, experts warn that, although progress has been made in treating the infection, HIV continues to remain a lethal infection for most people. Hence, education is the key to changing attitudes and lifestyles and, thus, preventing the contraction of HIV. Furthermore, society must understand that athletes are not a distinct population; they are as susceptible as anyone else to HIV.

Risk of HIV Infection and Modes of Transmission

Research indicates great difficulty in determining the actual risk of infection with HIV. Whether one acquires the virus depends on several factors. These include the individual's degree of susceptibility (everyone differs), mode of transmission, duration of the person's direct contact with the virus, strength of the dose of infection, and degree of resistance to the virus. Furthermore, lifestyle, such as sexual behaviors and sexual hygiene, can be related to the spread of the virus.

While HIV is found in almost all body fluids (such as blood, semen, vaginal and cervical secretions, breast milk, saliva, tears, urine, feces, cerebrospinal fluid, and sweat), transmission readily occurs only through the exchange of blood, semen, and vaginal and cervical secretions. The following three modes of transmission account for most cases of HIV infection in the United States (National Institute of Allergy and Infectious Diseases 1994):

• Sexual transmission: Unprotected sexual contact with an infected person transmits the virus. The presence of a concomitant sexually transmissible infection (STI), such as herpes, syphilis, chlamydia, or gonorrhea, makes an individual more susceptible to infection with HIV.
• Blood-to-blood transmission: Sharing of contaminated needles and syringes used for injecting drugs carries a high risk of HIV infection. The use of heat-treatment techniques to destroy HIV in blood products and routine screening of the blood supply before a transfusion (since 1985) have greatly reduced the risk of acquiring HIV through these means. Accidental transmission of HIV through

contaminated needle sticks and other medical equipment does not commonly occur anymore.

• Perinatal transmission (mother-to-fetus/infant transmission): An infected woman can transmit HIV to her unborn child during the pregnancy and to her newborn during delivery or after birth. The risk of transmission is estimated to be about 25%. Initiating treatment with AZT during pregnancy decreases the risk of perinatal transmission from 25% to 8.3% (Legg and Minkoff 1996).

Although many have speculated about the possible transmission of HIV through saliva and sweat, such transmission modes have not been proven to be possible. "To date there are no documented cases of HIV transmission in the United States from saliva, tears, or human bites" (Kell and Jenkins 1998). Calabrese and Kelly (1989) already showed that sweat, the most common bodily fluid exchanged between athletes, is not considered a risk factor for HIV transmission among athletes (see also Wormser et al. 1992). Other research studies conducted with health care personnel, including nurses, doctors, and dentists, did not provide sufficient evidence that HIV can be contracted through contact with saliva (Mertens 1995).

Incidence of HIV Infection in Sport

The possibility of HIV transmission in sport settings is often raised, especially when the media focus on a celebrity athlete infected with HIV. An analysis of the available epidemiological data about transmission of HIV clearly indicates the absence of a documented case of HIV transmission occurring within the sport setting (American Academy of Pediatrics 1992; Brown et al. 1994; Calabrese et al. 1993; World Health Organization 1989). Athletes who have been infected with HIV, to date, have contracted the virus outside the sport setting, mostly as a result of their lifestyles. Yet, this issue has raised considerable concern among athletes, coaches, sport organizations, and the general public.

Only one report indicates a possible transmission of HIV in sport. In 1989, two Italian soccer players collided and sustained head wounds. One player had contracted HIV from intravenous drug use; the other had previously tested negative for HIV but was later found to be HIV positive. Since no tests were conducted at the time of the head injury during the soccer match, the origin of the contracted HIV infection remains unknown. "Presently the medical community maintains with confidence that there are no known cases of HIV transmission occurring on a field of play" (Kell and Jenkins 1998; see also Torre et al. 1990).

In 1991, the U.S. Olympic Committee released a detailed report about the transmission of infectious agents during athletic competition. The report reiterated that no case of HIV transmission through sport has ever been documented. The riskiest sports for transmission of HIV and other blood-borne agents are clearly the bloodiest sports: boxing, wrestling, and tae kwon do (McGrew et al. 1993). Other collision sports such as football and ice hockey and contact sports such as basketball and soccer provide opportunities for open bleeding wounds to occur, providing a theoretical possibility of HIV transmission. Note that though certain sports can theoretically transmit HIV, no documented case of such transmission has occurred thus far.

The only case of HIV transmission that has occurred in a physical contest, *not a sporting contest,* occurred in Britain. "It involved a vicious punch-up during a wedding reception in London where . . . the participants 'rearranged each other's faces'" (Gray 1992). The article stated that one fighter transmitted HIV to the other. According to the president of the medical council of FIBA, the international basketball federation, "There is no evidence that similar transmission has occurred during a sporting event" (Gray 1992).

Nevertheless, several studies have analyzed the potential risk that HIV-positive athletes may pose when participating in sport, mainly contact sports. Brown et al. (1994) observed professional football players from 11 teams of the National Football League (NFL) during 155 regular-season games from September through December 1992. They observed 575 injuries of which 72 (12.5%) were lacerations. They then calculated the frequencies of bleeding injuries in association with athletic and environmental factors. Using these data, information about transmission of HIV in other circumstances, and HIV prevalence, the authors estimated the risk of transmission of HIV during football games. They calculated the risk to be less than one infection per 85,647,821 game contacts. Based on their data, the authors extrapolated that the probability of a single HIV transmission during an NFL season would be estimated to be 0.017, i.e., a transmission may occur less than once in 58.6 seasons. The current NFL policy does not require bleeding football players to leave the field. In the heat of the contest, "A punch is lightning quick and a tackle or a body check is extremely fast, making exposure time minute. Thus, the opportunity of contracting HIV during sports is quite minimal, but there is always some risk" (Kell and Jenkins 1998).

In another risk study of high school and college sports (Mueller and Cantu 1990), 36 football players were involved in fatal injuries. In other sports such as soccer, gymnastics, track, wrestling, and baseball, 12 fatal and 136 serious injuries occurred. Clearly, athletes are far more likely to suffer injuries or be killed on the playing field than to contract HIV through sport.

A study conducted in 1992 of 548 responding National Collegiate Athletic Association (NCAA) institutions (out of 860 surveyed) revealed that 35 (6%) had established policies about the participation of HIV-positive athletes, and 15 others had restricted participation in some way. Six of the institutions banned HIV-positive athletes from participating in any sport, while nine banned them only from selected sports such as ice hockey or wrestling (McGrew et al. 1993). These studies clearly reflect the major concerns the public *and* people in the sporting world, such as sport administrators, athletic trainers, and athletes, have in regard to HIV transmission, particularly for contact sports.

Consequently, even though the risk of HIV transmission in sport is highly unlikely, many voices advocate mandatory testing for all athletes, since the risk is not zero. However, several problems are associated with mandatory HIV testing. These include the high probability of false negative and false positive test results as well as issues regarding the right to privacy.

Testing for HIV Infection

Since an individual infected with HIV in its early stages may be asymptomatic, the diagnosis is made primarily by testing the individual's blood for the presence of antibodies to the virus. Antibodies are proteins produced by the body that are specific to each infectious agent. Blood-borne antibodies to HIV reach detectable levels in about one to three months following infection. At times, however, they may not be detected for as long as six months after infection. The period from the time of contact with HIV to the detection of antibodies to HIV in the blood is known as the window period. When an individual is in the window period, the HIV antibody test result will be negative while the person, if truly infected, can continue to transmit the virus to others through risky behaviors. Testing during the window period accounts for one of the most common reasons individuals receive a falsely negative HIV antibody test result (National Institute of Allergy and Infectious Diseases 1994).

An individual can undergo anonymous testing, where the testing personnel and test site do not know a person's identity. An individual can also opt for confidential testing, where only the health care provider knows the person's identity. Some NCAA-affiliated institutions and state sport organizations, such as the Nevada Boxing Association, have instituted mandatory testing as a precondition for participation in their institutional sports activities. In mandatory testing, an individual has to undergo HIV antibody testing if he or she wishes to participate in sport.

However, restricting HIV-positive athletes from participating in sport seems inadvisable (Volkwein, Sankaran, and Bonsall 1996). Restricting athletes from sport in order to prevent possible HIV transmission would probably not hold up in court. Since courts have already decided that discrimination against HIV-positive people in the work force is illegal, the same would probably apply to athletes. Excluding HIV-positive athletes from sport is probably illegal (see chapter 9).

Furthermore, numerous studies have shown that participation in sport is especially beneficial to the HIV-positive person. It helps to strengthen the immune system and thus to fight the disease; that is, exercise may actually help to stall the active onset of AIDS (LaPerriere et al. 1990; Rigsby et al. 1992) (see chapter 3). Consequently, mandatory testing of all athletes for HIV is impractical and inadvisable. The World Health Organization (WHO) has found no medical reason to screen athletes (World Health Organization 1992).

Guidelines to Minimize the Risk of Infection

Since no vaccine prevents infection with HIV, the focus of prevention has been to avoid risky behaviors that place an individual at risk of infection. These risky behaviors include participating in unprotected sexual intercourse and sharing contaminated needles and syringes. The Centers for Disease Control (CDC) has formulated guidelines called universal precautions to reduce the risk of transmission of HIV through exposure to body fluids. Organizations such as the National Athletic Trainers' Association have developed guidelines for dealing with blood-borne pathogens. Their members can use these guidelines to reduce the risk of transmission of HIV (National Athletic Trainers Association 1995) (see chapter 4 for further information).

Conclusion and Recommendations

An analysis of the available epidemiological data about transmission of HIV clearly indicates the absence of a documented case of HIV transmission occurring within the sport setting. Even though the risk of HIV transmission in sport is highly unlikely, the risk is not zero. Individuals will most likely contract HIV through lifestyle and not through sport participation and subsequent injuries. In addition, regular exercise has been proven to be very beneficial to people infected with HIV (see chapter 3). Thus, no reason exists to exclude any athlete from sport or to mandate HIV testing for all athletes before entering athletic contests. At the present time, athletic trainers should educate athletes and coaches to prevent the spread of HIV by practicing safe athletics. They should reinforce the establishment of rules and guidelines sensible for all parties involved and not discriminate against HIV-positive people participating in sport.

Recommendations to guard against HIV infection of others in sport are simple. First, educate all athletes about HIV and possible transmission. Second, encourage physicians to counsel the HIV-infected athletes, informing them of their responsibilities not to expose others to unnecessary risk of transmission. Third, make all athletes aware that the athletic program allows HIV-infected athletes to take part in sport. Fourth, make HIV testing available to all athletes who want to be tested. Fifth, use universal precautions when dealing with blood, scrapes, and open wounds. Although many sport organizations mandate regular testing for HIV, testing may not be necessary to protect the health and safety of the noninfected athletes, teammates, and medical personnel. Since testing is not an effective measure against the spread of HIV among athletes due to false test results, it should not be made mandatory.

References

American Academy of Pediatrics. (1992). American academy of pediatrics policy statement: Human immunodeficiency virus acquired immunodeficiency syndrome (AIDS) in the athletic setting. *The Physician and Sports Medicine, 20* (5), 189–91.

Brown, L.S., Phillips, R.Y., Brown, C.L., Knowlan, C., Castle, L., & Mover, J. (1994). HIV/AIDS policies and sports: The National Football League. *Medicine and Science in Sports and Exercise, 26,* 403–07.

Calabrese, L.H., Haupt, H., Hartman, L., & Strauss, R. (1993). HIV and sports, what is the risk? *The Physician and Sports Medicine, 21* (6), 173–80.

Calabrese, L.H., & Kelly, D. (1989). AIDS and athletics. *The Physician and Sports Medicine, 17* (1), 127–32.

Gray, C. (1992). AIDS becomes a sports issue. *Canadian Medical Association Journal, 146* (8), 1437–38.

Kell, R., & Jenkins, A. (1998). HIV transmission and sports: Realities and recommendations. *Strength and Conditioning*, February, 58–61.

LaPerriere, A., Antoni, M., Schneidermann, N., Ironson, G., Klimas, N., Caralis, P., & Fletcher, M.A. (1990). Exercise intervention attenuates emotional distress and natural killer cell decrements following notification of positive serologic status for HIV-1. *Biofeedback and Self-Regulation, 15* (3), 229-242.

Legg, J.J., & Minkoff, H.S. (1996). Vertical transmission: Now preventable. *Patient Care, 30,* 160–63.

McGrew, C., Randall, W., Schneidwind, K., & Gikas, P. (1993). Survey of NCAA institutions concerning HIV/AIDS policies and universal precaution. *Medicine and Science in Sports and Exercise, 25,* 917–21.

Mertens, T. (1995). HIV-Infektionsrisiko beim sport. In: Bundesministerium fuer Gesundheit (ed.) *Handbuch "Sport und HIV-Infektion."* Baden-Baden, Germany: Nomos, 41–48.

Mueller, F., & Cantu, R. (1990). Catastrophic injuries and fatalities in high school and college sports, fall 1982 - spring 1988. *Medicine and Science in Sports and Exercise, 22,* 734–741.

National Athletic Trainers Association. (1995). Bloodborne pathogens guidelines for athletic trainers. *Journal of Athletic Training , 30* (3), 203–04.

National Institute of Allergy and Infectious Diseases. (1994). *HIV infection and AIDS.* Bethesda, MD: United States Department of Health and Human Services, Public Health Service, December 2.

Rigsby, L., Dishman, R., Jackson, A., Maclean, G., & Raven, R. (1992). Effects of exercise training on men seropositive for the human immunodeficiency virus-1. *Medical Science and Sport Exercise, 24* (1), 6–12.

Torre, D., Sampietro, C., Ferraro, G., Zaroli, C., & Speranza, I. (1990). Transmission of HIV-1 infection via sports injuries [Letter]. *Lancet , 335* (8697), 1105.

United Press International. (1989). *Views on minorities tied to AIDS attitudes.* March 24.

United Press International. (1991). *Attitude toward AIDS victims depends on sexual preference.* August 27.

USA Today. (1996). *Morrison's cavalier attitude worries doctors.* August 26.

Volkwein, K.A.E., Sankaran, G., & Bonsall, D. (1996). Bleeding wounds and the threat of HIV: The role of athletic trainers. *Athletic Therapy Today, 1* (1), 38–41.

World Health Organization Consensus Statement: Consultation on AIDS and Sports. (1992). *Journal of the American Medical Association, 267* (10), 1312.

World Health Organization, in Collaboration with the International Federation of Sports Medicine. (1989). *Consensus Statement from Consultation on AIDS and Sports.* Geneva, Switzerland: WHO.

Wormser, G., Bittker, S., & Forester, G. (1992). Absence of infectious human immunodeficiency virus type 1 in "natural" eccrine sweat. *Journal of Infectious Diseases, 165* (1), 115–18.

CHAPTER 2

Epidemiology, Immunology, and Clinical Spectrum of HIV and AIDS

Gopal Sankaran

West Chester University of Pennsylvania

This chapter focuses on the epidemiology, immunology, and clinical spectrum of the human immunodeficiency virus (HIV) infection. It includes a discussion of the virus's structure and the alterations to the normal immune mechanism. This chapter also addresses the epidemiology of HIV infection in the United States based on person, place, and time distribution as well as the natural history and clinical spectrum of HIV infection. It explains the available testing methods to detect HIV infection, problems of false positive and false negative results with testing, and testing alternatives (confidential and anonymous). This chapter also addresses management of HIV infection and AIDS and the prognosis for those who are HIV positive. Consult the glossary to clarify the meaning of scientific terminology used in chapters 2 and 3.

Epidemiology of HIV Infection

This section will address the epidemiology (distribution and determinants) of HIV/AIDS both from a global and a national perspective. Reports of a new syndrome (a group of signs and symptoms) designated as acquired immunodeficiency syndrome (AIDS) were reported among gay men in June 1981 in the United States. Since then, the disease has become a global pandemic affecting more than 190 countries. More than 2.3 million cases were reported to the World Health Organization (WHO) by the end of 1997 (Quinn 1996; UNAIDS and WHO 1997). However, the reported cumulative number of AIDS cases represents just the tip of the iceberg. Inadequate health infrastructure and information systems have led to gross underdiagnosis and underreporting of cases, particularly in developing nations. When taking into account inadequacies in data, an estimated 11.7 million deaths due to AIDS are estimated to have occurred in adults and children since the known beginning of the epidemic (UNAIDS and WHO 1997).

The WHO has estimated that about 30 million persons throughout the world are infected with HIV. This number is expected to increase to 40 million by the year

2000. The majority of those infected likely live in developing nations (UNAIDS and WHO 1997). The *Report on the Global HIV/AIDS Epidemic* (UNAIDS and WHO 1997) indicated that about 16,000 new HIV infections occurred each day in 1997. According to the same report, many of the 30 million people currently infected with HIV may die within the next decade.

Total new HIV infections occurring in 1997:   5.8 million
Estimated number of people living with HIV/AIDS: 30.6 million
Projected estimate of people living with HIV by 2000:   40 million
Total AIDS deaths in 1997:   2.3 million
Estimated total AIDS deaths since the beginning of the epidemic: 11.7 million

In spite of this alarming background, rapid strides have been made in the understanding of the causative organism (the HIV), the disease process, the detection of HIV infection in humans, and the management of those infected with HIV. More recent estimates (Holmberg 1996) indicate that about 650,000 to 900,000 persons living in the United States are infected with HIV. Since an accurate distribution of HIV infection in the world (or in the United States) is not known, the author will present the epidemiology of AIDS in the United States. Noteworthily, at the 5th Conference on Retroviruses in February 1998, the suggestion was made that mandatory reporting of all new HIV infections to the Centers for Disease Control and Prevention (CDC) would provide more accurate statistics. If implemented nationwide, physicians and researchers would have a better description of the status of HIV in the United States (Klaus and Grodesky 1998b).

As of December 1997, the cumulative number of AIDS cases in the United States reported to the CDC was 641,086. Cases occurring in males—538,703—represent 84% of the total. Cases occurring in females—102,383—represent 16% of the total. From January 1981 to December 1997, adult and adolescent cases of AIDS totaled 633,000 (98.7%). During the same period, a total of 8,086 cases (1.3% of total reported cases) were reported in children (that is, persons under age 13 at the time of diagnosis) (CDC 1997a) (table 2.1).

In the United States, the first cases of AIDS were reported to the CDC in 1981. In the 15 years thereafter, over 500,000 cases have been reported (CDC 1997b).

Table 2.1   Age and Gender Distribution of Cumulative Number of AIDS Cases Reported in the United States as of December 1997

Age Group	Male	Female	Total
Adults and adolescents	534,532	98,468	633,000
Children (<13 years at the time of diagnosis)	4,171	3,915	8,086
Total	538,703	102,383	641,086

Source: Centers for Disease Control and Prevention 1997a

During this time frame, in late 1987 and again in late 1992, the AIDS surveillance case definition (effective January 1,1993) was expanded substantially (CDC 1987; 1992). Two factors prompted the changes in surveillance definition. First, knowledge gained about the natural history of HIV had increased. Second, the clinical management of HIV-positive individuals needed to maintain consistency (CDC 1995). So, it is worthwhile to consider the temporal changes in the reporting of AIDS cases during these three time periods: 1981–1987, 1988–1992, and 1993–1995. Noteworthily, of the cumulative AIDS cases in the United States, 50,352 (10%) were reported to the CDC during 1981–1987; 203,217 (41%) during 1988–1992; and 247,741 (49%) during 1993–late 1995 (CDC 1995).

During 1981–1987, females constituted 8% of the reported AIDS cases. During 1993–October 1995, they formed 18% of the total reported AIDS cases. The proportion of cases among injecting drug users (IDUs) during the same time periods changed from 17% to 27%. Cases attributed to heterosexual transmission during the same time periods increased from 3% to 10%. However, cases among men who have sex with men showed a decline from 64% to 45% (CDC 1995).

During 1981–1987 and 1993–October 1995, the proportion of cases among whites declined from 60% to 43%. During the same time frame, the proportion among African Americans and Hispanics showed an increase. For African Americans, AIDS cases increased from 25% to 38% and for Hispanics from 14% to 18% (CDC 1995).

During 1996 in the United States, the rate of new AIDS cases per 100,000 was 115.3 among African Americans, 55.8 among Hispanics, 16.2 among whites, 14.1 among Native Americans/Native Alaskans, and 7.5 among Asians/Pacific Islanders. This indicates a disproportionately greater burden of the disease among African Americans and Hispanics in the country (CDC 1997b).

According to CDC HIV/AIDS surveillance data (1997a), as of December 1997, the top 10 states or territories that reported the highest number of AIDS cases among their residents were New York, California, Florida, Texas, New Jersey, Puerto Rico, Illinois, Pennsylvania, Georgia, and Maryland. The top 10 metropolitan areas reporting the highest number of AIDS cases, as of December 1997, were New York City; Los Angeles; San Francisco; Miami; Washington, DC; Chicago; Houston; Philadelphia; Newark; and Atlanta (CDC 1997a).

From 1981–1987, the Northeast and West accounted for the majority (38.8% and 26.9%, respectively) of total reported AIDS cases. However, during 1988–1992 and 1993–October 1995, the largest number of reported cases were in the South. This geographic area also accounted for the largest proportionate increase of reported cases (31%) (CDC 1995). The number of reported cases in smaller metropolitan statistical areas (MSAs) (areas with a population of 50,000–499,000) and non-MSAs (rural areas) has increased. During 1993–October 1995 in the South and Midwest, both MSAs and non-MSAs have shown higher proportions of cases among adolescents and young adults (aged 13–29 years) as compared to the Northeast and West (CDC 1995).

Chapter 1 discusses, in detail, how HIV is and is not transmitted. Note that since the HIV antibody test became available in 1984, all blood and blood products in the United States have been routinely screened for HIV since May 1985. This has resulted in a decrease in the proportion of cases of AIDS linked to blood transfusions (2.6% in 1981–1987 to 1.0% in 1993–October 1995) (CDC 1995).

Immunology and HIV Infection

Two classes of white blood cells (WBC) direct the normal immune system in a healthy adult. The first class, lymphocytes, respond to a specific invading foreign organism. The second class includes cells such as macrophages, eosinophils, natural killer cells, and mast cells that nonspecifically attack invading foreign organisms. Lymphocytes are of two types: B-lymphocytes and T-lymphocytes.

B-lymphocytes secrete soluble proteins called antibodies into the bloodstream. These attach to the specific antigens encountered. Antigens are parts of the invading organism that elicit an antibody response. One foreign organism can have several different antigenic parts and, consequently, elicit the formation of several different antibodies. After binding to the antigen, the antibody signals other cells of the immune system to join the fight. This constitutes *humoral immunity,* as it encompasses the production of antibodies that circulate in the bloodstream (Alcamo 1997; Fan, Conner, and Villarreal 1998; Schindler 1990).

T-lymphocytes, on the other hand, make proteins known as receptors. These receptors are on the surfaces of T-lymphocyte cells and are not released into the bloodstream. These cells then target specific antigens and bind to them. This constitutes *cell-mediated immunity* (CMI), as the cells themselves bind with the specific antigens. The T-lymphocytes are predominantly of two types: T-killer cells (also known as cytotoxic T-cells) and T-helper cells. T-killer cells are further categorized into T-suppressor cells and natural killer cells. T-helper cells have CD4+ protein markers on their surfaces and are also known as CD4+ cells. T-killer cells have CD8+ protein markers and, hence, are known as CD8+ cells. Laboratory tests now make it possible to identify the CD4+ and CD8+ proteins. This allows physicians and researchers to estimate the amount of T-helper and T-killer lymphocytes in a person's blood (Alcamo 1997; Fan et al. 1998; Schindler 1990). This is referred to as a CD4+ count (the number of T-helper cells) or, alternatively, a CD8+ count (the number of T-killer cells).

The function of the two types of T-lymphocytes differ. The T-killer cells directly bind to cells carrying a foreign antigen and kill them. The T-helper cells interact with B-lymphocytes and T-killer cells, facilitating their response to invading antigens. T-helper cells thus play a critical role in both humoral and cell-mediated immunity. In humoral immunity, they provide the necessary signal to a B-lymphocyte that has already bound to an antigen. This causes the B-lymphocyte to divide and secrete antibodies that neutralize the antigen. When a deficiency of T-helper cells occurs, the T-killer cells cannot divide after successfully binding to their specific antigens. This occurs in AIDS and results in both impaired immunologic protection against opportunistic infections and development of certain cancers (Alcamo 1997; Fan et al. 1998; Miralles 1996).

Molecular Structure of HIV

HIV is a member of the Lentivirinae family of retroviruses. This family of viruses is often associated with silent infections with long latency. This type of infection has the capability to affect the central nervous system (CNS) (Levy 1993). Retroviruses have a fairly simple molecular structure. HIV has three major parts. The first, an outer envelope, contains the major proteins of HIV (gp120 and g41). The second part, an inner core, has four proteins (p24, p7, p17, and p9). Inside the core lies two copies of single-stranded ribonucleic acid (RNA). HIV has three main genes in its structure—gag, env, and pol. The gag gene encodes the core nuclear capsule of the virus. The env gene encodes the surface proteins of the virus. The pol gene encodes the enzyme reverse transcriptase, which gives the virus the unique ability to synthesize deoxyribonucleic acid (DNA) using its own RNA as a template (Levy 1993).

After entering the human body, the reverse-transcribed viral DNA (called the *provirus*) incorporates into the genome of the WBC or lymphocyte. The provirus is then able to replicate itself using the host's cellular machinery. Thus, HIV successfully makes use of human cells to replicate itself. In addition, HIV has six other genes (vif, vpu, vpr, tat, rev, and nef) that possibly enable the virus to establish an inactive state in some infected host cells and then allow for reactivation at later times (Alcamo 1997; Fan et al. 1998; Miralles 1996).

Effects of HIV on the Immune System and Immunologic Markers

Soon after HIV enters the body through the various modes of transmission (as described in chapter 1), it widely disseminates. It predominantly enters the lymph node tissue distributed at different sites in the body. The immune response mounted by the body and trapping of the virus in lymph nodes partially blocks initial entry and dissemination of HIV in the new host (Fauci 1996). The initial strong host immune response results in a marked decrease in the number of viral particles found in peripheral blood. Unfortunately, the body does not eliminate all the viral particles. This sets the stage for chronic, persistent viral replication in the host, exemplified by the chronic nature of HIV infection and AIDS (Fauci 1996). Three possible theories explain the incomplete clearing of the virus during the primary immune response. First, the magnitude of the immune response may be inadequate. Secondly, some components of the immune response may be missing during the initial stage of HIV infection. Thirdly, it is also possible that HIV may have mechanisms to escape the immune response (Pantaleo and Fauci 1995).

In the body, HIV targets those T-helper cells and macrophages that display the CD4+ surface protein and then attaches itself to those cells. HIV infects and causes the death of T-helper cells, depleting the body of these cells. HIV may not kill macrophages but may establish a dormant infection in them. From its base in macrophages, HIV generates and releases new viral particles into the bloodstream. These new viruses then continue the process of infecting previously uninfected T-helper cells and other macrophages (Fan et al. 1998; Miralles 1996).

Lymph nodes are the major reservoir for and site of persistent viral replication. This has been noted both early in the course of HIV infection and during the period of clinical latency when the CD4+ count is only moderately reduced (Pantaleo et al. 1993). In the early stage of HIV infection, the lymph nodes of persons with progressive AIDS are activated and become enlarged (lymphadenopathy). These enlarged lymph nodes could occur in different areas of the body (such as the neck, axilla, and inguinal region), warranting a diagnosis of generalized lymphadenopathy. Lymph nodes have a complex structure. They contain various types of cells and spaces to hold lymph, a type of body fluid. Many viral particles (virions) are found trapped in the germinal centers of lymph nodes in the extracellular (outside the cell) space on follicular dendritic cells (a type of cell in a lymph node). This facilitates continuing immune stimulation. It also allows for possible infection of T-helper cells that reside in or are migrating through the lymph nodes. This, in turn, leads to the ultimate destruction of lymphoid tissue and culminates in suppression of the immune system. So, at the beginning of HIV infection, the process of viral replication is matched by the production of T-helper cells and T-killer cells by the infected host. At later stages of the HIV infection, viral replication overtakes the capacity of the immune system to produce T-helper cells (Fauci 1996).

By understanding the molecular structure of HIV and how it adversely affects the immune system (immunopathogenesis), researchers have developed suitable laboratory tests that help monitor the progression of HIV infection and AIDS. Initially, investigations included counting the number of T-helper and T-killer cells and determining their comparative ratio. In contrast, current techniques allow physicians to estimate the total number of virus particles throughout the course of the disease. Viral culture, polymerase chain reaction (PCR), plasma HIV RNA, and p24 antigen are some of the testing methods currently available for monitoring the various stages of HIV infection and AIDS (Hutton 1996).

Clinical Spectrum of HIV Infection

The natural history of a disease refers to the stages of an infection when the infection is left untreated. Most of the natural history of HIV infection is based on data obtained from homosexual males enrolled in various clinical studies in the late 1970s and the 1980s. As knowledge about HIV, its life cycle, and the immunopathogenesis has evolved, so has the natural history of this condition.

Pantaleo, Graziosi, and Fauci (1993) divided the clinical course of HIV infection into three phases. The first phase is primary infection, which is present in about 50–70% of HIV-infected individuals as a nonspecific, mononucleosis-like clinical syndrome of variable severity. The second phase involves the period of clinical latency, which may be long (median—10 years). During the third phase, AIDS becomes clinically apparent. It is characterized by persistent constitutional symptoms and/or increased susceptibility to opportunistic infections and/or certain cancers.

John Bartlett (1997) recently classified the natural history of HIV infection into the following seven stages (see table 2.2). The first four are viral transmission, primary HIV infection, seroconversion, and a clinical latent period with or without persistent generalized lymphadenopathy (PGL). The fifth stage involves early symptomatic HIV infection. This was previously reported as AIDS-related complex (ARC). The CDC in its revised 1993 classification has categorized these as B symptoms. The sixth and seventh stages are AIDS and advanced HIV disease. According to the 1987 CDC criteria and revised 1993 CDC criteria, a diagnosis of AIDS requires a CD4+ count <200/mm^3. Advanced HIV disease, however, is characterized by a CD4+ cell count <50/mm^3.

Table 2.2   Stages of HIV Infection and CD4+ Cells

---

1. Viral transmission (CD4+ cell count is normal; about 1000/mm^3)

2. Primary HIV infection

3. Seroconversion

4. Clinical latent period with or without persistent generalized lymphadenopathy (PGL) (average rate of decline of CD4+ cells is about 50/mm^3 per year)

5. Early symptomatic HIV infection (CD4+ cells around 500/mm^3)

6. Acquired immunodeficiency syndrome (AIDS) (CD4+ cells <200/mm^3)

7. Advanced HIV disease (CD4+ cells <50/mm^3)

Used with permission, from J.G. Bartlett, 1997, Natural History and Classification. In *Medical Management of HIV Infection*. Retrieved October 15, 1998 from the World Wide Web: **http://www.hopkins-aids.edu/publications/index_pub.html**

Viral Transmission

As mentioned in Chapter 1, viral transmission occurs through unprotected sexual intercourse with a person infected with HIV, exposure to blood infected with HIV, or perinatal transmission. Perinatal transmission includes infection of the unborn through the placenta, infection of the newborn at the time of vaginal delivery, or postpartum infection of the child through breastfeeding (Hutton 1996).

Primary HIV Infection

Primary HIV infection is also called acute HIV infection or acute seroconversion syndrome. The incubation period from the time of exposure to the onset of symptoms and signs is usually 2–4 weeks, but it may take as long as 6 weeks (Pedersen et al. 1989). Symptoms and signs are reported in about 50–90% of individuals who provide a history of the usual risky behaviors that put them at risk for HIV transmission (Fox, Eldred, and Fuchs 1987; Pedersen et al. 1989; Tindall et al. 1988). The symptoms often mimic acute infectious mononucleosis (mono). They typically include fever, lymphadenopathy, sore throat, rash on the face and trunk and at times over the extremities, lesions in the mucous membranes of the mouth or genitals, myalgia (muscular pain), arthralgia (joint pain), diarrhea, headache, nausea and vomiting, hepatosplenomegaly (enlargement of the liver and the spleen), and thrush. Infection with HIV is seldom considered or recognized at this stage, even if symptomatic persons seek medical help (Bartlett 1997).

Diagnosis at this stage of the illness is best established by demonstration of a high level of HIV in the blood. Two tests, p24 antigen and plasma HIV RNA, with negative or indeterminate HIV serology in a person with typical clinical features should alert the health care provider to consider this diagnosis (Clark et al. 1991). Acute symptoms and signs last about 1–4 weeks (and average 2 weeks), and then the person recovers. A dramatic decline in plasma HIV RNA levels is noted with recovery (Bartlett 1997).

Seroconversion

This is the stage when the HIV-infected person tests positive with a laboratory test used to detect HIV antibodies in the serum. When a test shows the presence of HIV antibody, a person is said to have seroconverted. Seroconversion usually takes place about 6–12 weeks following exposure to the virus. Over 95% of HIV-positive people seroconvert within about six months following HIV transmission (Bartlett 1997). The time from exposure to HIV to seroconversion is often referred to as the window period (Fan et al. 1998).

Early HIV Disease

The period beginning with seroconversion and continuing for the following six months refers to the early HIV disease stage of the disease. During this time, considerable variation in CD4+ count and virus count or burden is noted (Bartlett 1997). At about 6 months after seroconversion, the viral burden in the patient establishes a set point that shows minimal variation during years of follow-up (Bartlett 1997; Mellors, Rinaldo, Gupta, White, Todd, and Kingsley 1995).

Asymptomatic Infection

During this phase of the infection, the person is clinically without symptoms or signs except for enlarged lymph nodes involving at least two noncontiguous sites other than inguinal nodes (Bartlett 1997). This is called persistent generalized lymphad-enopathy or PGL. During this phase, contrary to earlier belief, high rates of HIV production occur with destruction of T-helper cells daily. About one-third of viral load in the body is turned over daily, which means that one in three viral particles are removed from the body each day. This is accompanied by a rapid turnover of T-helper cells, averaging 6–7% of the total body T-helper cells. Therefore, all T-helper cells in the body are replaced every 15 days (Ho, Neumann, Perelson, Chen, Leonard, and Markowitz 1995; Perelson, Neumann, Markowitz, Leonard, and Ho 1996; Wei et al. 1995).

Early Symptomatic HIV Infection

Early symptomatic HIV infection (used to be called ARC) is referred to as B conditions by the CDC. This phase includes conditions that are more likely to be found in the presence of HIV infection and tend to be more severe. Examples include thrush, persistent and/or recurrent vaginal candidiasis (a type of yeast infection), cervical dysplasia (abnormal changes in cervical tissue), oral hairy leukoplakia (white thickened patches with a tendency to break up and the potential to become malignant), peripheral neuropathy (functional and structural changes in the peripheral nerves affecting nerve conduction), and constitutional symptoms (generalized, affecting the whole body) (Bartlett 1997). By revised CDC definition (effective January 1, 1993), these illnesses by themselves do not qualify as AIDS-indicator conditions (CDC 1992).

Acquired Immunodeficiency Syndrome (AIDS)

The currently followed CDC surveillance definition of AIDS (effective January 1, 1993) includes all the AIDS-indicator diseases in the 1987 version plus recurrent bacterial pneumonia, pulmonary tuberculosis, and invasive cervical cancer. The definition also includes all persons with a CD4+ count of <200/mm^3 (CDC 1987, 1992). The median time from the onset of severe immunosuppression (defined as a CD4+ count <200mm^3) to an AIDS-defining illness (using 1987 CDC criteria) is about 12–18 months in individuals not receiving any treatment. In contrast, severe immunosuppression is delayed by 9–10 months in those receiving AZT (Bartlett 1997).

Advanced HIV Infection

This stage characterizes those persons with HIV infection whose CD4+ count has fallen to <50 mm^3. Median survival time for persons in this stage is 12–18 months. Death due to HIV-related complications occur in this group (Bartlett 1997).

Progression of AIDS

The average time from HIV seroconversion to death is about 10 years in the absence of treatment (Bartlett 1997). The median time from seroconversion to AIDS (by 1987 CDC definition) was about 7 years for transfusion recipients, 8–12 years for gay men, 10 years for IDUs, and 10 years for hemophiliacs. No differences occurred in the rate of progression based on gender, race, and risk category if adjusted for quality of care (Bartlett 1997). However, the treating health care provider's experience in AIDS care appears to influence survival (Kitahata, Koepsell, Deyo, Maxwell, Dodge, and Wagner 1996; Paauw, Wenrich, Curtis, Carline, and Ramsey 1995). Age, too, is an important variable in the progression of disease. For patients aged 16–24 at seroconversion, the median time from seroconversion to AIDS was 15 years. In contrast, for those aged 35 or older at seroconversion, the median time until AIDS was 6 years. Extensive individual variations exist in the progression of AIDS (Bartlett 1997).

The number of virus particles and CD4+ count are important variables for progression of the disease. A higher number of virus particles and a steeper T-helper cell decline denote a rapid progression of the disease with resultant poor prognosis (Mellors et al. 1996). (The average rate of decline of T-helper cells is about 50/mm^3 per year.) Preservation of lymph node architecture is associated with delayed progression of the illness (Fauci 1996). T-helper cell loss may accelerate in later stages of the illness as viral load increases (McMichael and Phillips 1997). According to a recent report by Vlahov et al. (1998), plasma HIV viral load independently and in combination with T-helper cell count measurements were useful in determining disease progression.

According to Fauci et al. (1996), fewer than 5% of HIV-infected persons showed no indication of infection progression and have stable levels of T-helper cells. The lymph nodes in long-term nonprogressors retained their architectural integrity and preserved their stromal environment (normal connective tissue forming the ground substance in the lymph nodes). These individuals also showed much lower levels of trapped virions in their lymphatic tissue. Correlates with delayed progression include: low viral burden, well-preserved structural layout of lymph node cells, nonsynctium-inducing HIV (that is, the infection does not lead to merging of cellular contents), and increased T-killer cells activity (Bartlett 1997). Long-term nonprogressors are now being studied to find out why their immune system is able to protect them so long from the destruction usually induced by HIV (Dean et al. 1996).

Testing and Diagnosis of HIV Infection

Diagnosis of HIV infection should include a thorough risk assessment, detailed medical history, and clinical examination followed by laboratory tests. Currently available tests to detect HIV infection include HIV antibody tests (enzyme-linked immunosorbent assay [ELISA] and western blot [WB]), HIV p24 antigen test, HIV RNA, HIV PCR, and HIV culture. The most widely available tests to detect HIV infection are the HIV antibody tests. The CDC (1992) has recommended an algorithm for testing for HIV infection. All tests need to be administered with informed consent and should include pretest and posttest counseling. A sample of blood from the individual should be tested twice using the ELISA test. If the test results are positive, then they need to be confirmed by a confirmatory test, such as the WB test. If the WB test also yields a positive result, then the person is informed that he or she is infected with HIV.

The current generation of ELISA tests, when combined with the WB test, have a very high sensitivity and specificity (over 99.5% each). However, the tests are not 100% accurate. False positives and false negatives can happen. False negatives can occur during the window period. This problem can be minimized by retesting six months after the first test (Fan et al. 1996). A false positive test can result from contamination of the sample and cross-reactivity due to certain other immunosuppressive conditions such as lymphomas, sarcoidosis, and so forth.

As of 1996, the Food and Drug Administration (FDA) has approved an oral, fluid-based test for checking antibodies to HIV. The OraSure testing system, an oral HIV test, consists of a specially treated cotton pad attached to a nylon stick and a vial containing a preservative solution. Collecting the specimen is fairly simple. The pad is placed between the lower cheek and gum, rubbed back and forth until moistened, then left in place for a couple of minutes. This test is equivalent to the serum test in its accuracy but is safer and easier to use (Malamud 1997). Non-HIV medical conditions and oral diseases do not appear to influence the test results.

A person who wishes to know his or her HIV status can participate in any of the following three testing options:

• Anonymous testing. Currently, many testing centers in several states offer anonymous testing. The person who wishes to undergo an HIV antibody test is not required to provide any personal identifying information such as name, address, phone number, and social security number. The person is provided with a code, and the same code is attached to the blood sample. The person can obtain the test result by contacting the testing center and referencing the provided code. As an advantage, this option provides complete anonymity to the person who undergoes testing. Unfortunately, the person who undergoes anonymous testing is responsible to seek counseling; the testing center has no way to trace the person to offer counseling.

• Confidential testing. In this form of testing, the person who undergoes testing is counseled by a health care provider prior to testing and also receives posttest counseling from the provider. Thus, the health care providers will know the identity of the individual undergoing testing. While this approach ensures the availability of counseling services, breach of confidentiality is a potential risk.

• Home-testing kits. Anonymous testing for HIV infection is now possible at home through the availability of self-use kits such as Access and Confide. Clear instructions allow the test to be carried out in the anonymity of one's own home. The individual obtains test results by calling a toll-free number and using the code provided with the test kit. These toll-free numbers also allow the caller to obtain on-line counseling and referral services.

Treatment of HIV Infection

The management of HIV infection and its complications involves team effort—the person with HIV infection, his or her family, close friends, a primary care provider, and specialists, as needed. A holistic approach is required with due attention paid to emotional, mental, physical, and spiritual needs of the person with HIV infection. This section addresses only the medical management of HIV infection.

Until late 1986, only one antiretroviral drug, AZT or zidovudine, had been approved by the FDA for treatment of HIV infection. This drug is a nucleoside analogue and acts by inhibiting the activity of reverse transcriptase, an enzyme needed by HIV to transform its own RNA material into DNA as a step toward its replication. Since 1987, the FDA has approved four more nucleoside analogues for use against HIV infection. These include didanosine (ddI), zalcitabine (ddC), stavudine (d4T), and lamivudine (3TC) (Ungvarski 1997). Using one nucleoside analogue alone (referred to as *monotherapy*) induced viral resistance, the ability of HIV to replicate and infect cells in the presence of the drug. Adding another nucleoside analogue resulted in a more sustained action against HIV and delayed the troublesome drug resistance.

In late 1995, the FDA approved a new group of antiretroviral drugs effective against the enzyme protease in HIV. Protease is instrumental in breaking up a larger viral protein into the smaller proteins necessary for assembling infectious viral particles. These new sets of antiretroviral drugs act by inhibiting the protease enzyme, and hence are called *protease inhibitors.* Use of these drugs results in the formation of a noninfectious virus. This group of drugs offers additional ammunition to attack another point in the life cycle of HIV. As of December 1996, three protease inhibitors had been approved for use by the FDA. These include saquinavir (Invirase), indinavir (Crixivan), and ritonavir (Norvir) (Deeks et al. 1997; Ungvarski 1997). A fourth drug, nelfinavir (Viracept), is available through an expanded-access program (Deeks, Smith, Holodniy, and Kahn 1997). At present, the licensed protease inhibitors include saquinavir in two forms (Invirase and Fortovase), indinavir (Crixivan), ritonavir (Norvir), and nelfinavir (Viracept) (Klaus and Grodesky 1998a).

Currently, physicians and researchers recommend the use of combination therapies (using a cocktail approach) to prevent the emergence of resistant strains of HIV. This usually includes a three-drug regimen including two nucleoside analogue reverse transcriptase inhibitors and a protease inhibitor. The double protease inhibitor combination of saquinavir and ritonavir is also effective (Gulick 1998). Detailed guidelines for antiretroviral therapy have been made available by the International AIDS Society—USA Panel (Carpenter et al. 1997). Proper dosing and continuous treatment are also recommended to delay the development of resistance. The aggressive use of combination therapies can lead to a tremendous decline in viral load. These drugs have been so effective that the possibility of viral eradication has been raised (Carpenter et al. 1997; Deeks et al. 1997). However, the experience with these newer drugs is too limited to warrant such optimism.

The downside to such optimistic pronouncements is the cost of combination therapies. The total annual cost of combination therapy plus the associated monitoring for viral load may be well over $10,000 per year assuming no major toxicity occurs (Deeks et al. 1997). The costs need to be weighed against the potential decrease in health care costs among users who are able to delay or avoid complications and hospitalizations. Such an analysis is feasible if long-term studies could be conducted in the absence of drug resistance. The previous estimate of $119,000 as the lifetime cost of treating a person with HIV from the time of infection until death (Hellinger 1993) is under revision since the advent of highly effective but expensive protease inhibitors. The lifetime cost of treating HIV infection and AIDS may appear to be high. However, a number of medical interventions widely accepted to be standard treatment procedures and considered to be worth their costs are also expensive: $26,000 for coronary artery bypass graft surgery, $46,000 for renal dialysis, and $154,000 for hypercholesterolemia treatment (Tengs et al. 1995 as cited in Rose 1998). The cost of HIV therapies (including prophylaxis regimens), relative to the benefit they extend to quality of life, conform well to the accepted range of other medical care. Hence, timely access to these cost-effective HIV therapies for all patients with HIV infection can prove beneficial by adding quality years to their lives (Rose 1998).

Recently, interleukin-2 (IL-2) administered to persons with AIDS resulted in noticeable increases in CD4+ counts in a magnitude and for a duration not seen in previous clinical trials with antiretroviral agents. The use of immunomodulator therapy (capable of modifying or regulating immune functions), such as IL-2, to boost the immune response provides a viable alternative to viral suppression by blocking replication of the virus (Kovacs et al. 1996).

Prospects of Prevention Through Vaccines

Johnston (1997) provided an excellent rationale for developing a vaccine that can be employed to prevent HIV infection. Vaccination is perhaps one of the most cost-effective ways of dealing with an infectious disease such as AIDS. When using pharmacological agents, physicians and recipients must pay careful attention to cost, drug resistance, tolerance, side effects, and toxicity. Most persons throughout the globe infected with HIV can hardly afford the currently available medications. Prevention, in most instances, is cheaper than treatment even if the costs of treatment decrease in the near future. This makes the prospect of prevention through vaccines an attractive alternative. Vaccines, once tested and accepted for human use, could be mass produced and delivered. They are generally easy to administer and efficient. They provide lasting benefits and could be unlinked from human behaviors (the major reason for becoming infected with HIV) (Johnston 1997).

Considerable challenges, however, hinder the development of a vaccine against HIV infection. Immunization must occur prior to onset of sexual activity or injecting drug use and afford long-term protection. The vaccine must be affordable by developing nations where most of the HIV infections in the late 1990s and next decade are expected to occur. The vaccine may need to protect against multiple strains of the virus. No established correlates of protection exist. All of these factors must also contend with several other problems in HIV vaccine development. First, U.S. manufacturers currently show diminished interest in vaccine production due to safety concerns. This has led to slowed development of vaccines. Also, their interest has diminished because their opportunity to make profit is limited. Mass vaccination will be needed in poorer nations who may not be able to pay for the vaccine. Second, technical difficulties are related to the lack of an ideal animal model, rapid mutation of HIV after infection, and difficulty in inducing mucosal immunity. This mucosal immunity is required to protect individuals in whom HIV gains entry through the vaginal or rectal mucosa. Due to these hurdles, the arrival of a safe, simple, inexpensive, effective vaccine in the market in the near future is unlikely (Francis 1995; Johnston 1997).

However, reasons for optimism exist. Vaccination has proven to be successful against other viral diseases such as measles, mumps, poliomyelitis, and hepatitis A and B. Experimental vaccines have protected monkeys (macaques) and apes (chimpanzees) from simian immunodeficiency virus (SIV). Candidate vaccines have induced a strong immune response in humans. Adults infected with attenuated HIV remain healthy. Lowering the viral load by using antiretroviral drugs provides a clinical benefit, and mucosal transmission of HIV occurs relatively inefficiently (Johnston 1997). All of these factors lead to a renewed call and effort for a vaccine to prevent and contain HIV infection.

Current prospects for an HIV vaccine include preparations employing the envelope of HIV or core proteins, peptide vaccines, designs based on synthetic particles, prime-boost vaccines based on recombinant canarypox or vaccinia viruses, and nucleic acid or naked DNA vaccines (Haynes 1996; Johnston 1997). The worldwide spread of HIV needs to be stopped at all costs, and only a vaccine can accomplish that.

Conclusion and Recommendations

Since the identification of AIDS in 1981, more than half-a-million people have developed AIDS in the United States. Over three-fifths of those diagnosed with AIDS have already died. The global picture is even gloomier. However, rapid strides are being made in understanding the progression of HIV infection and how to treat it. Delaying the progression of HIV infection is possible in the 1990s by using the newly available antiretroviral treatments. Current research about AIDS indicates that the disease may very well become a chronic condition that is treatable but not curable (like diabetes or hypertension) in the next decade, as compared to it being a killer disease in the 1980s. Vaccine development has accelerated, but the availability of a vaccine to the public before the end of the century seems remote.

Risk reduction and behavior modification are effective strategies in reducing HIV acquisition and transmission in specific population groups. These strategies need to be continued and strengthened while the world waits for a vaccine to prevent HIV infection and a cure for the resultant disease. Every person must become aware of the types of behaviors that place one at risk of contracting HIV. Any person who feels that he or she is possibly infected with HIV should undergo voluntary testing for the infection as soon as possible so that early diagnosis and treatment can be initiated. Additional information about HIV and AIDS is available through national and state AIDS hotlines. Refer to the section "A Guide to Resources for HIV/AIDS" in the book. All participants (both amateurs and professionals) in sport must know the ways by which they can avoid contracting and transmitting HIV. They should also practice behaviors that promote prevention and control of this global problem.

References

Alcamo, I. E. (1997). *AIDS: The Biological Basis*. Dubuque, IA: Brown.

Bartlett, J. G. (1997). Natural History and Classification. In *Medical Management of HIV Infection*. The Johns Hopkins AIDS Service: Medical Mgt. of HIV. Retrieved October 15, 1998 from the World Wide Web: **http://www.hopkins-aids.edu/publications/index_pub.html**

Carpenter, C. C. J., Fischl, M. A., Hammer, S. M., Hirsch, M. S., Jacobsen, D. M., Katzenstein, D. A., Montaner, J. S. G., Richman, D. D., Saag, M. S., Schooley, R. T., Thompson, M. A., Vella, S., Yeni, P. G., & Volberding, P. A. (1997). Antiretroviral therapy for HIV infection in 1997: Updated recommendations of the international AIDS society—USA Panel. *Journal of the American Medical Association, 277* (24), 1962-69.

Centers for Disease Control and Prevention (CDC). (1987). Revision of the CDC surveillance case definition for acquired immunodeficiency syndrome. *Morbidity and Mortality Weekly Report, 36* (Suppl 1), 3S-14S.

Centers for Disease Control and Prevention (CDC). (1992). 1993 revised classification system for HIV infection and expanded surveillance case definition for AIDS among adolescents and adults. *Morbidity and Mortality Weekly Report, 41* (RR-17), 1-19.

Centers for Disease Control and Prevention (CDC). (1995). First 500,000 AIDS cases — United States, 1995. *Morbidity and Mortality Weekly Report, 44* (45), 849-53.

Centers for Disease Control and Prevention (CDC). (1997a). *HIV/AIDS Surveillance Report, 9* (2), 3-43. Atlanta, GA: U. S. Department of Health and Human Services, Public Health Service.

Centers for Disease Control and Prevention (CDC). (1997b). Update: Trends in AIDS incidence, deaths, and prevalence—United States, 1996. *Morbidity and Mortality Weekly Report, 46* (8), 165-73.

Clark, S. J., Saag, M. S., Decker, W. D., Campbell-Hill, S., Roberson, J. L., Veldkamp, P. J., Kappes, J. C., Hahn, B. H., & Shaw, G. M. (1991). High titers of cytopathic virus in plasma of patients with symptomatic primary HIV-1 infection. *New England Journal of Medicine, 324* (14), 954-60.

Dean, M., Carrington, M., Winkler, C., Huttley, G. A., Smith, M. W., Allikmets, R., Goedert, J. J., Buchbinder, S. P., Vittinghoff, E., Gomperts, E., Donfield, S., Vlahov, D., Kaslow, R., Saah, A., Rinaldo, C., & Detels, R. (1996). Genetic restriction of HIV-1 infection and progression to AIDS by a deletion allele of the CKR5 structural gene. *Science, 273* (5283), 1856-1862.

Deeks, S. G., Smith, M., Holodniy, M., & Kahn, J. O. (1997). HIV-1 protease inhibitors: A review for clinicians. *Journal of the American Medical Association, 277* (2), 145-153.

Fan, H., Conner, R. F., & Villarreal, L. P. (1998). *AIDS: Science and Society* (2nd ed.). Boston: Jones and Bartlett.

Fauci, A. S. (1996). Immunopathogenic mechanisms of HIV infection. NIH Conference. *Annals of Internal Medicine, 124* (7), 654-663.

Fox, R., Eldred, L. J., & Fuchs, E. J. (1987). Clinical manifestations of acute infection with human immunodeficiency virus in a cohort of gay men. *AIDS, 1* (1), 35-38.

Francis, D. P. (1995). Why AIDS vaccine development is taking longer than it should. *Current Issues in Public Health, 1* (1), 181.

Gulick, R. M. (1998). Editorial: HIV treatment strategies: Planning for the long term. *Journal of the American Medical Association, 279* (12), 957-58.

Haynes, B. F. (1996). HIV vaccines: Where we are and where we are going. *Lancet, 348* (9032), 933-937.

Hellinger, F. J. (1993). The lifetime cost of treating a person with HIV. *Journal of the American Medical Association, 270* (4), 474-478.

Ho, D. D., Neumann, A. U., Perelson, A. S., Chen, W., Leonard, J. M., & Markowitz, M. (1995). Rapid turnover of plasma virions and CD4+ lymphocytes in HIV-1 infection. *Nature, 373* (6510), 123-126.

Holmberg, S. D. (1996). The estimated prevalence and incidence of HIV in 96 large US metropolitan areas. *American Journal of Public Health, 86* (5), 642-54.

Hutton, N. (1996). Health prospects for children born to HIV-infected women. In R. R. Faden & N. E. Kass (Eds.), *HIV, AIDS and Childbearing: Public Policy, Private Lives* (pp. 63-77). New York: Oxford University Press.

Johnston, M. I. (1997). HIV vaccines: Problems and prospects. *Hospital Practice, 32* (5), 125-140.

Kitahata, M. M., Koepsell,T. D., Deyo, R. A., Maxwell, C. L., Dodge, W. T., & Wagner, E. H. (1996). Physician's experience with the acquired immunodeficiency syndrome as a factor in patients' survival. *New England Journal of Medicine, 334* (11), 701-06.

Klaus, B. D., & Grodesky, M. J. (1998a). HIV news: Drug interactions and protease inhibitor therapy in the treatment of HIV/AIDS. *The Nurse Practitioner, 23* (2), 104-06.

Klaus, B. D., & Grodesky, M. J. (1998b). HIV news: News from the 5th conference on retroviruses and opportunistic infections. *The Nurse Practitioner, 23* (4), 117-27.

Kovacs, J. A., Vogel, S., Albert, J. M., Falloon, J., Davey, R. T., Walker, R. E., Polis, M. A., Sponner, K., Metcalf, J. A., Baseler, M., Fyfe, G., & Lane, C. H. (1996). Controlled trial of interleukin-2 infusions in patients with the human immunodeficiency virus. *New England Journal of Medicine, 335* (18), 1350-56.

Levy, J. A. (1993). Pathogenesis of human immunodeficiency virus infection. *Microbiological Review, 57* (1), 183-89.

Malamud, D. (1997). Oral diagnostic testing for detecting human immunodeficiency virus-1 antibodies: A technology whose time has come. *The American Journal of Medicine, 102* (Suppl 4A), 9-14.

McMichael, A. J., & Phillips, R. E. (1997). Escape of human immunodeficiency virus from immune control. *Annual Review of Immunology, 15*, 271-96.

Mellors, J. W., Kingsley, L. A., Rinaldo, C. R., Jr., Todd, J. A., Hoo, B.S., Kokka, R. P., & Gupta, P. (1995). Quantitation of HIV-1 RNA in plasma predicts outcome after seroconversion. *Annals of Internal Medicine, 122* (8), 573-579.

Mellors, J. W., Rinaldo, C. R., Gupta, P., White, R. M., Todd, J. A., & Kingsley, L. A. (1996). Prognosis in HIV-1 infection predicted by the quantity of virus in plasma. *Science, 272* (5265), 1167-70.

Miralles, G. (1996). Virology and pathogenesis of HIV. In Bartlett, J. A. (Ed.), *Care and Management of Patients With HIV Infection* (pp.1-38). Research Triangle Park, NC: Glaxo Wellcome, Inc.

Paauw, D. S., Wenrich, M. D., Curtis, R., Carline, J. D., & Ramsey, P. G. (1995). Ability of primary care physicians to recognize physical findings associated with HIV infection. *Journal of the American Medical Association, 274* (17), 1380-82.

Pantaleo, G., Graziosi, C., Demarest, J. F., Butini, L., Montroni, M., Fox, C. H., Orenstein, J. M., Kotler, D. P., & Fauci, A. S. (1993). HIV infection is active and progressive in lymphoid tissue during the clinically latent stage of the disease. *Nature, 362* (6418), 355-58.

Pantaleo, G., Graziosi, C., & Fauci, A. S. (1993). The immunopathogenesis of human immunodeficiency virus infection. *New England Journal of Medicine, 328* (5), 327-35.

Pantaleo, G., & Fauci, A. S. (1995). New concepts in the immunopathogenesis of HIV infection. *Annual Review of Immunology, 13*, 487-512.

Pedersen, C., Lindhart, B. O., Jensen, B. L., Lauritzen, E., Gerstoft, J., Dickmeiss, E., Gaub, J., Scheiber, E., & Karlsmark, T. (1989). Clinical course of primary HIV infection. Consequences for subsequent course of infection. *British Medical Journal, 299* (6692), 154-157.

Perelson, A. S., Neumann, A. U., Markowitz, M., Leonard, J. M., & Ho, D. D. (1996). HIV-1 dynamics *in vivo*: Virion clearance rate, infected cell life-span, and viral generation time. *Science, 271* (5255), 1582-1586.

Quinn, T. C. (1996). Global burden of the HIV pandemic. *Lancet, 348* (9020), 99-106.

Rose, D. N. (1998). Editorial: AIDS drug regimens that are worth their costs. *Journal of the American Medical Association, 279* (2), 160-61.

Schindler, L. W. (1990). *Understanding the Immune System*. (NIH Publication No. 90-529, pp. 3-20). Bethesda, MD: U.S. Department of Health and Human Services, Public Health Service, National Institutes of Health.

Tengs, T. O., Adams, M. E., Pliskin, J. S., Safran, D. G., Siegel, J. E., Weinstein, M. C., & Graham, J. D. (1995). Five-hundred life-saving interventions and their cost-effectiveness. *Risk Analysis, 15* (3), 369-90.

Tindall, B., Barker, S., Donovan, B., Barnes, T., Roberts, J., Kronenberg, C., Gold, J., Penny, R., & Cooper, D. (1988). Characteristics of the acute clinical illness associated with human immunodeficiency virus infection. *Archives of Internal Medicine, 148* (4), 945-49.

UNAIDS & WHO. (1997). *Report on the Global HIV/AIDS Epidemic*. Retrieved October 15, 1998 from the World Wide Web: **http://www.unaids.org/highband/ document/epidemio/report97.html**

Ungvarski, P. J. (1997). Update on HIV infection. *American Journal of Nursing, 97* (1), 44-51.

Vlahov, D., Graham, N., Hoover, D., Flynn, C., Bartlett, J. G., Margolick, J. B., Lyles, C. M., Nelson, K. E., Smith, D., Holmberg, S., & Farzadegan, H. (1998). Prognostic indicators for AIDS and infectious disease death in HIV-infected injection drug users: Plasma viral load and CD4+ cell count. *Journal of the American Medical Association, 279* (1), 35-40.

Wei, X., Ghosh, S. K., Taylor, M. E., Johnson, V. A., Emini, E. A., Deutsch, P., Lifson, J. D., Bonhoeffer, S., Nowak, M. A. , Hahn, B. H., Saag, M. S., & Shaw, G. M. (1995). Viral dynamics in human immunodeficiency virus type 1 infection. *Nature, 373* (6510), 117-122.

CHAPTER 3

HIV, Exercise, and Immune Function

Bente Klarlund Pedersen

National University Hospital in Copenhagen, Denmark

Many individuals claim that regular exercise increases resistance to infections such as the common cold (Fitzgerald 1988; Nash 1987). On the other hand, anecdotal reports from athletes and their coaches indicate that hard training is associated with increased respiratory tract infections. Today, epidemiological evidence exists that supports the anecdotal impression (Nieman and Henson 1994). Clearly, moderate physical activity enhances the function of the immune system and may be somewhat responsible for an exercise-related reduction in illness. In contrast, research has repeatedly shown that intense exercise causes inhibition in immune system function during the recovery phase following it (Hoffman-Goetz and Pedersen 1994; Pedersen 1997).

Given that both acute and chronic exercise modulates the immune system, determining how exercise influences the immune system in immunosuppressed patients, such as those infected with the human immunodeficiency virus (HIV), is important. This chapter describes the effects of acute and chronic exercise on the immune system in HIV seropositive individuals.

The Immune Defect in HIV Infection

The natural course of HIV infection is dominated by a progressive immunosuppression leading to the development of AIDS. Severe opportunistic infections and malignant diseases occur in the majority of infected individuals (Fauci 1988; Rosenberg and Fauci 1990). The primary immunologic defect in individuals infected with HIV is a depletion of T-helper cells (Fauci 1988). The number and percentage of T-helper cells have been established as strong and reliable predictors of the progression to AIDS and death (Phillips, Pezzoti, Cozzi-Lepri, and Rezza 1994). However, the number of T-helper cells (CD4+ count) does not thoroughly describe the immune defect caused by HIV. T-helper cells can be broadly categorized into a CD45RA+ subset and a CD45RO+ subset. Within the T-helper cell population during HIV infection, an early loss of CD45RO+ cells is followed by an increased loss of CD45RA+ cells. In advanced infection, this is highly predictive of death (Ullum, Lepri, Victor, Skinhoj, Phillips, and Pedersen 1997).

In the population of T-killer (CD8+) cells, early increases in numbers and in expression of activation markers have been related to a poorer outcome. The functional capacity of lymphocytes can be evaluated by lymphocyte proliferation, which can occur either spontaneously or be stimulated by mitogens or antigens. A defective proliferative response has been detected early in HIV infection and has been related to a poorer prognosis (Hofmann et al. 1989).

Furthermore, the disease suppresses the function of natural killer (NK) cells and lymphokine-activated killer (LAK) cells early in its progress (Ullum, Gotzsche, Victor, Dickmeiss, Skinhoj 1995). Note that both NK and LAK cells are part of the cell-mediated immune system. The NK cells are apparently the primary defense mechanism against tumor cells, which the body recognizes as foreign. They can also attack microbes and infected cells. However, NK cells are less specialized than LAK cells. The lymphokines released by the T-helper cells stimulate LAK to multiply rapidly. The LAK cells then move from the lymph nodes into the circulation, where they target the microbe-infected cells (be they infected with bacteria, viruses, fungi, or protozoa) and destroy them. Thus, immune-cell activation occurs early in HIV infection. Markers of such activation are useful for predicting the progression to AIDS in individuals.

The Effects of Acute Exercise on HIV-Positive Individuals

Exercise alters the concentrations of lymphocyte subpopulations, proliferative responses, as well as NK and LAK cell functions in normal, healthy individuals. HIV impairs these immune parameters. When taking these factors together, it is obviously important to determine if exercise influences the immune system differentially in HIV-positive and HIV-negative subjects.

Ullum et al. (1994) performed a study on acute exercise (cycling for one hour at 75% of $\dot{V}O_2$max) designed to determine the extent HIV-infected individuals can mobilize immunocompetent cells to the blood in response to physical exercise. Immunocompetent cells are those cells able to mount a normal immune response. The study included eight asymptomatic men infected with HIV and eight HIV-negative controls who cycled for one hour at 75% of $\dot{V}O_2$max. The HIV-positive subjects did not have AIDS or an AIDS-related complex and had a CD4+ cell count of 200–500 cells/μl.

The level of T-helper cells in the circulation has prognostic value for predicting the development of acquired immunodeficiency syndrome (AIDS) in HIV-infected patients. It also has prognostic value for predicting mortality resulting from complications of HIV infection in AIDS (Safai et al. 1985; Taylor, Afrasiabi, Fahey, Korns, Weaver, Mitsuysau 1986). However, increases in the concentration and percentage of T-helper cells in response to treatment may not always reflect a better prognosis (Concorde 1994; Kovacs et al. 1995).

Researchers and physicians have debated about which immunologic marker to use: the absolute number or the percentage of T-helper cells. Taylor, Fahey, Detels, & Giorgi (1989) showed that the percentage of T-helper cells had slightly greater prognostic significance and had slightly less variability in repeated measurements. The CD4+ count, but not the percentage of T-helper cells compared with the relative number of other lymphocytes, changes in response to acute exercise. This offers one explanation of the variability in the absolute numbers of T-helper cells. Furthermore, it also strengthens the idea that the percentage of T-helper cells is preferable to the number of T-helper cells in monitoring HIV-positive patients.

Interestingly, HIV-positive subjects possess an impaired ability to mobilize neutrophils (a type of white blood cell) and cells mediating NK cell activity. Furthermore, only control, HIV-seronegative persons showed increased LAK cell activity in the blood in response to exercise, whereas HIV-positive subjects did not (Ullum et al. 1994). Exercise is accepted as a model of physical stress. The study of acute exercise suggests that HIV-positive subjects, although only moderately immunosuppressed, possess an impaired ability to generate unspecific immunity toward microbial agents in response to various physical stimuli.

Another study (Rohde, Ullum, Palmo, Halkjaer-Kristensen, Newsholme, and Pedersen 1995) researched the effects of short exercise sessions on the immune response in HIV-positive and HIV-negative participants. T-helper cells from HIV-positive individuals were less likely to divide, grow, and increase in number (known as *proliferative response*) than those T-helper cells from HIV-negative persons. The mechanisms behind such a defective proliferative response are poorly understood. This defective response may occur because HIV-infected persons have an impaired hormone response, defective NK cells, or an overall lower number of T-helper cells (Doweiko 1993). The previous discussion indicates that the immune suppression, though minimal, in HIV-positive individuals does produce an important impairment in their ability to fight infections by other microbes.

The Effect of Chronic Exercise on the Immune System in HIV-Positive Individuals

Most studies have described chronic exercise or training as having no effect on lymphocyte proliferation in healthy, HIV-negative individuals (Nieman et al. 1995; Pedersen, Tvede, Christensen, Klarlund, Kragbak, and Halkjaer-Kristensen 1989; Tvede, Steensberg, Baslund, Halkjaer-Kristensen, and Pedersen 1991). One study showed that chronic exercise enhanced resting levels of the CD4+ count in this group of individuals (LaPerriere et al. 1994). In addition, most studies found no effect on concentrations or percentages of T-helper cells in HIV-negative subjects (Barnes et al. 1991; Nieman et al. 1995; Pedersen et al. 1989; Tvede et al. 1991). However, trained HIV-negative athletes reportedly have enhanced resting levels of NK cell function compared with untrained subjects (Hoffman-Goetz and Pedersen 1994; Nieman 1996).

Only a few controlled studies have researched the effect of chronic exercise on the immune system in HIV-positive subjects. Rigsby, Dishman, Jackson, Maclean, and Raven (1992) performed a controlled, randomized study. It included 19 HIV-positive subjects in stages II, III, and IV according to the Centers for Disease Control and Prevention (CDC) classification system. Stage II refers to HIV-positive, asymptomatic individuals. Stage III refers to HIV-positive individuals with persistent, generalized lymphadenopathy. Stage IV refers to HIV-positive individuals who manifest other diseases such as constitutional disease, neurological disease, secondary infections, secondary cancers, or other conditions attributed to HIV infection or immunosuppression. The subjects performed bicycle exercise training for 12 weeks. The study included 18 HIV-positive individuals who did not exercise to act as controls. Immune monitoring included flow cytometry analysis of lymphocyte subpopulations. Although training induced significant increases in neuromuscular strength and cardiorespiratory fitness, no significant effects occurred in the CD4+ count or other lymphocyte subpopulations in the HIV-positive individuals who exercised.

LaPerriere, Antoni, Schneiderman, Ironson, Caralis, and Fletcher (1990) performed a similar randomized, controlled training study. Their study included 10 HIV-positive subjects who performed bicycle exercise training for 45 minutes three times a week for 10 weeks. The study also included HIV-positive control subjects who did not train. The researchers initially reported that the CD4+ count, the CD56+ NK cell count, and the NK cell activity measured per CD56+ cell in whole blood did not change as a result of training. However, a later review article by LaPerriere, Fletcher, Antoni, Klimas, Ironson and Schneiderman (1991) reported increases in the CD4+ count and in the number of T-helper cells (CD4+ subtype CD4+45RA+) using the same exercise protocol and number of subjects. Birk and MacArthur (1994) included five HIV-positive subjects in a one-year training study. MacArthur, Levine, and Birk (1993) studied six HIV-positive subjects, CDC stage IV, who performed 24 weeks of training. Training had no effect on the CD4+ count in either of the studies.

One study, unfortunately, does not report the number of dropouts (LaPerriere et al. 1990). However, other studies reported one of five (20%) (Birk and MacArthur 1994), four of 23 (17%) (Rigsby et al. 1992), and 19 of 25 (76%) (MacArthur, Levine, and Birk 1993) dropouts. Clinical deterioration in some patients is probably a major cause of the high dropout rates reported in training studies including HIV-positive patients. Thus, although Rigsby et al. (1992) did not find differences between the training group and the control group regarding the number of subjects who dropped out or died, it cannot be excluded that HIV-positive subjects dropped out because exercise training worsened their condition. These dropouts therefore constitute a very important group clinically. If training induces an immunologic and clinical deterioration in some patients who then dropped out of the training program, the results would be biased.

Some of the studies have shown an insignificant increase in CD4+ count in patients that train. Based on these results, researchers have concluded that training increases the CD4+ count in HIV-positive patients (LaPerriere et al. 1991). This is a very important conclusion since it could lead to the acceptance of physical training as a treatment for HIV infection. However, no study has been able to show, to the author's knowledge, any significant effect of training on the CD4+ count in HIV-infected patients. If patients with declining CD4+ counts drop out of the exercise regimen due to declining health, this could lead to a false impression of an increasing CD4+ count caused by physical training.

Recently, the ability to measure HIV-RNA in plasma has contributed to the understanding of the pathogenesis of HIV infection. Recent data demonstrate that a continuous, high replication of HIV leads to exhaustion of the vast proliferative capacity of the host's immune system. In other words, the destruction of the T-helper cells eventually exceed their replenishment (Ho, Neumann, Perelson, Chen, Leonard, and Markowitz 1995; Wei et al. 1995). The use of both CD4+ counts and plasma HIV RNA measurements to monitor HIV-infected patients has greatly added to the prognostic value of the isolated use of the CD4+ count for predicting progression of HIV infection.

In order to accept exercise as a treatment for HIV infection, exercise must be shown not only to increase CD4+ counts but also to reduce the viral load and the immunologic activation as expressed by plasma HIV-RNA and serum β_2-microglobulin. Furthermore, since HIV infection inhibits the function of the cellular immune response, a truly positive clinical effect of any treatment for HIV infection would also lead to increases in the functional capacity of the cellular immune system.

However, there are no studies on the effect of training on viral load as measured by plasma HIV-RNA. Also, no data exist that show a beneficial effect of chronic exercise or training on resting levels of lymphocyte proliferation and cytotoxic functions in HIV-positive individuals.

The Open Window Hypothesis

In essence, moderate and severe exercise of short duration enhance the immune system. Suppressed concentration of lymphocytes, suppressed NK and LAK cell activity, and decreased secretory IgA (a type of antibody) in mucosa follow only intense, long-duration exercise. Thus, after intense, long-duration exercise, the immune system is temporarily suppressed. This period has also been called the *open window* (Pedersen and Ullum 1994). During the open window, microbes—especially viruses—may invade the host and establish infections. One reason for the increased susceptibility to infections seen in elite athletes could be that this window of opportunity for pathogens is longer and the degree of immunosuppression is more pronounced. The author has previously suggested that severe immunosuppression may occur if athletes do not allow the immune system to recover but, instead, initiate a new bout of exercise while still immunosuppressed. Brines, Hoffman-Goetz, and Pedersen (1996) have recently suggested that neutrophils (a type of white blood cell) serve as a last line of defense. During the open window's immune suppression of lymphoid cells, neutrophils are being mobilized to plug these gaps. The removal of this backup system following extreme activity would be compatible with the increased frequency of upper respiratory tract infections that occur in athletes.

Regarding HIV seropositive subjects, it was shown (Ullum et al. 1994) that these subjects have an impaired ability to mobilize neutrophils to the blood during exercise. Thus, HIV-positive subjects have an impaired immune system when measured at rest and, furthermore, an impaired ability to mobilize neutrophils to the blood during exercise stress. Therefore, in theory, HIV-positive subjects may be more prone to enter the so-called open window of the immune system and may more easily acquire infections during the time of postexercise immunosuppression.

Conclusion and Recommendations

Although no systematic research is available regarding the effects of moderate exercise on the immune system of HIV-positive subjects, no reasons exist to think that moderate exercise detrimentally affects the immune system of HIV-infected individuals. Findings regarding the effect of chronic training on resting levels of the immune system in HIV-positive patients are not consistent. Therefore, the available amount of data do not allow the drawing of any strong conclusions regarding possible beneficial or detrimental effects of training, regardless of intensity and duration, on the immune system of HIV-positive subjects. Thus, any encouragement for HIV-positive patients to perform physical exercise relies on the positive effects of muscle strengthening and oxygen uptake and the psychological relief achieved in those patients able to participate in a training program.

References

Barnes, C.A., Forster, M.J., Fleshner, M., Ahanotu, E.N., Laudenslager, M.L., Mazzeo, R.S., Maier, S.F., & Lal, H. (1991). Exercise does not modify spatial memory, brain autoimmunity, or antibody response in aged F-344 rats. *Neurobiological Aging, 12* (1), 47–53.

Birk, T.J., & MacArthur, R.D. (1994). Chronic exercise training maintains previously attained cardiopulmonary fitness in patients seropositive for human immunodeficiency virus type 1. *Sports Medicine Training and Rehabilitation 5*, 1–6.

Brines, R., Hoffman-Goetz. L., & Pedersen, B.K. (1996). Can you exercise to make your immune system fitter? *Immunology Today, 17* (6), 252–54.

Concorde. (1994). MRC/ANRS randomised double-blind controlled trial of immediate and deferred zidovudine in symptom-free HIV infection. Concorde Coordinating Committee. *The Lancet, 343* (8902), 871–81.

Doweiko, J.P. (1993). Hematologic aspects of HIV infection. *AIDS, 7* (6), 753–57.

Fauci, A.S. (1988). The human immunodeficiency virus: Infectivity and mechanisms of pathogenesis. *Science, 239*, 617–22.

Fitzgerald, L. (1988). Exercise and the immune system. *Immunology Today 9* (11), 337-39.

Ho, D.D, Neumann, A.U., Perelson, A.S., Chen, W., Leonard, J.M., & Markowitz, M. (1995). Rapid turnover of plasma virions and CD4+ lymphocytes in HIV-1 infection [see comments]. *Nature, 373* (6510), 123–26.

Hoffman-Goetz, L., & Pedersen, B.K. (1994). Exercise and the immune system: A model of the stress response? *Immunology Today, 15* (8), 382–87.

Hofmann, B., Jakobsen, K.D., Odum, N., Dickmeiss, E., Platz, P., Ryder, L.P., Pedersen, C., Matthiesen, I.B., Bygbjerg, I.C., & Faber, V. (1989). HIV-induced immunodeficiency. Relatively preserved phytohemagglutinin as opposed to decreased pokeweed mitogen responses may be due to possibly preserved responses via CD2/phytohemagglutinin pathway. *Journal of Immunology, 142*, 1874–80.

Kovacs, J.A., Baseler, M., Dewar, R.J., Vogel, S., Davey, R.T., Jr., Falloon, J., Polis, M.A., Walker, R.E., Stevens, R., & Salzman, N.P. (1995). Increases in CD4+ T lymphocytes with intermittent courses of interleukin-2 in patients with human immunodeficiency virus infection. A preliminary study [see comments]. *New England Journal of Medicine, 332* (9), 567–75.

LaPerriere, A., Antoni, M.H., Ironson, G., Perry, A., McCabe, P., Klimas, N., Helder, L., Schneiderman, N., & Fletcher, M.A. (1994). Effects of aerobic exercise training on lymphocyte subpopulations. *International Journal of Sports Medicine, 15* (Supplement 3), S127–30.

LaPerriere, A., Antoni, M.H., Schneiderman, N., Ironson, G., Caralis, P., & Fletcher, M.A. (1990). Exercise intervention attenuates emotional distress and killer cell decrements following notification of positive serologic status for HIV-1. *Biofeedback and Self-Regulation, 15* (3), 229–42.

LaPerriere, A., Fletcher, M.A., Antoni, M.H., Klimas, N.G., Ironson, G., & Schneiderman, N. (1991). Aerobic exercise training in an AIDS risk group. *International Journal of Sports Medicine, 2* (Supplement 1), S53–57.

MacArthur, R.D., Levine, S.D., & Birk, T.J. (1993). Supervised exercise training improves cardiopulmonary fitness in HIV-infected persons. *Medicine and Science in Sports and Exercise, 25* (6), 684–88.

Nash, H.L. (1987). Can exercise make us immune to disease? *Physician and Sportsmedicine*, (1), 250-53.

Nieman, D.C., Brendle, D., Henson, D.A., Suttles, J., Cook, V.D., Warren, B.J., Butterworth, D.E., Fagoaga, O.R., & Nehlsen-Cannarella, S.L. (1995) Immune function in athletes versus nonathletes. *International Journal of Sports Medicine, 16* (5), 329–33.

Nieman, D.C., & Henson, D.A. (1994). Role of endurance exercise in immune senescence. *Medicine and Science in Sports and Exercise, 26* (2), 172–81.

Nieman, D.C. (1996). Prolonged aerobic exercise, immune response, and risk of infection. In L. Hoffman-Goetz (Ed.), *Exercise and Immune Function* (pp. 143–162). Boca Raton, FL: CRC Press.

Pedersen, B.K. (Ed.). (1997). *Exercise Immunology* (pp. 1–206). Austin, TX: R.G. Landes.

Pedersen, B.K., Tvede, N., Christensen, L.D., Klarlund, K., Kragbak, S., & Halkjaer-Kristensen, J. (1989). Natural killer cell activity in peripheral blood of highly trained and untrained persons. *International Journal of Sports Medicine, 10* (2), 129–31.

Pedersen, B.K., & Ullum, H. (1994). NK cell response to physical activity: Possible mechanisms of action. *Medicine and Science in Sports and Exercise, 26* (2), 140–46.

Phillips, A.N., Pezzoti, P., Cozzi-Lepri, A., & Rezza, G. (1994). CD4+ lymphocyte count as a determinant of the time from seroconversion to AIDS and death. Evidence from the Italian Seroconversion Study. *AIDS, 8* (9), 1299-1305.

Rigsby, L.W., Dishman, R.K., Jackson, A.W., Maclean, G.S., & Raven, P.B. (1992). Effects of exercise training on men seropositive for the human immunodeficiency virus-1. *Medicine and Science in Sports and Exercise, 24* (1), 6–12.

Rohde, T., Ullum, H., Palmo, J., Halkjaer-Kristensen, J., Newsholme, E.A., & Pedersen, B.K. (1995). Effects of glutamine on the immune system—influence of muscular exercise and HIV infection. *Journal of Applied Physiology, 79* (1), 146–50.

Rosenberg, Z.F., & Fauci, A.S. (1990). Immunopathogenic mechanisms of HIV infection: Cytokine induction of HIV expression. *Immunology Today, 11* (5), 176–80.

Safai, B., Johnson, K.G., Myskowski, P.L., Koziner, B., Yang, S.Y., Cunningham Rundles, S., Godbold, J.H., & Dupont, B. (1985). The natural history of Kaposi's sarcoma in the acquired immunodeficiency syndrome. *Annals of Internal Medicine, 103* (5), 744–50.

Taylor, J., Afrasiabi, R., Fahey, J.L., Korns, E., Weaver, M., & Mitsuysau, R. (1986). Prognostically significant classification of immune changes in AIDS with Kaposi's sarcoma. *Blood, 67* (3), 666–71.

Taylor, J.M., Fahey, J.L., Detels, R., & Giorgi, J.V. (1989). CD4+ percentage, CD4+ number, and CD4+:CD8+ ratio in HIV infection: Which to choose and how to use. *Journal of Acquired Immune Deficiency Syndrome, 2* (2), 114–24.

Tvede, N., Steensberg, J., Baslund, B., Halkjaer-Kristensen, J., & Pedersen, B.K. (1991). Cellular immunity in highly trained elite racing cyclists during periods of training with high and low intensity. *Scandinavian Journal of Medicine, Science, and Sports, 1*, 163–66.

Ullum, H., Gotzsche, P.C., Victor, J., Dickmeiss, E., Skinhoj, P., & Pedersen, B.K. (1995). Defective natural immunity: An early manifestation of human immunodeficiency virus infection. *Journal of Experimental Medicine, 182* (3), 789–99.

Ullum, H., Lepri, A.C., Victor, J., Skinhoj, P., Phillips, A.N., & Pedersen, B.K. (1997). Increased losses of CD4+CD4+5RA+ cells in late stage of HIV infection is related to increased risk of death: Evidence from a cohort of 347 HIV-infected individuals. *AIDS, 11* (2), 1479–85.

Ullum, H., Palmo, J., Halkjaer-Kristensen, J., Diamant, M., Klokker, M., Kruuse, A., LaPerriere, A., & Pedersen, B.K. (1994). The effect of acute exercise on lymphocyte subsets, natural killer cells, proliferative responses, and cytokines in HIV-seropositive persons. *Journal of Acquired Immune Deficiency Syndrome, 7* (11), 1122–33.

Wei, X., Ghosh, S.K., Taylor, M.E., Johnson, V.A., Emini, E.A., Deutsch, P., Lifson, J.D., Bonhoeffer, S., Nowak, M.A., & Hahn, B.H. (1995). Viral dynamics in human immunodeficiency virus type 1 infection. *Nature, 373* (6510), 117–22.

CHAPTER 4

HIV, the Game Official, and Control and Prevention

Corrie J. Odom
Kessler Memorial Hospital Rehabilitation Services, New Jersey

Greg Strobel
Lehigh University, Pennsylvania

Little information can be found about exposure to or governing policy regarding human immunodeficiency virus (HIV) and game officials. Professional journals and periodicals related to health, recreation, athletics, sports medicine, and officiating lack a·discussion about the risk of transmission of HIV and other blood-borne pathogens to the officials in charge of the game. More striking is the lack of information addressing the role of the game officials in preventing the transmission of HIV to themselves or to other participants.

In college and high school athletics, the game officials do not typically become involved with handling the bleeding athletes. However, the officials are at risk for exposure to blood. A referee or umpire may be called upon or feel it is his or her duty to assist with a bleeding athlete or blood spill in the absence of qualified medical personnel such as a certified athletic trainer, physician, emergency medical technician, paramedic, or school nurse. Even when the game officials are not charged with attending to a bleeding athlete or the surroundings contaminated by a blood spill, the officials should still be educated in the use of universal precautions.

Organizing and coordinating sporting events incorporates the sharing of responsibilities by administrative and support personnel. However, once the clock starts, the ball goes up, or the starting gun fires, the game officials assume an omnipotent role. To execute their duties, game officials must preside over all aspects of play governed by the existing rules for a particular sport. Recent additional rules require the officials to assume primary responsibility for identifying the bleeding player, stopping play to remove the involved player from the game, and determining if bleeding has been properly controlled prior to the athlete reentering the game (Federation Rule Changes for 1994 1994; National Association of Intercollegiate Athletics (NAIA) 1993; National Collegiate Athletic Association (NCAA) Committee on Competitive Safeguards and Medical Aspects of Sports 1993).

Game officials, whether certified, rated, paid, or volunteers, have a very important role in preventing the potential transmission of HIV as a result of blood exposure during an athletic contest. Indeed, as the world moves toward the 21st century, involvement in sport presents new and potentially lifesaving challenges for those who preside over the rules of competition. This chapter will critically assess the educational aspects of officiating as they relate to the awareness and prevention of HIV transmission.

Risk of HIV Transmission

Researchers and physicians widely accept that the risk of transmitting HIV during athletic competition is minimal (American Academy of Pediatrics [AAP] Policy Statement 1992; American Orthopedic Society for Sports Medicine [AOSSM] and the American Academy of Sports Medicine [AASM] 1995; Calabrese, Haupt, Hartman, and Strauss 1993; Hamel 1992; Johnson 1992; Mast, Goodman, Bond, Tavero, and Drotman 1995; Seltzer 1993). Yet, the prevalence and incidence of HIV infection in teenagers and young adults warrants prudent action by all persons participating in sport events where injuries and contact are imminent and probable. While contact and collision sports present a higher risk of blood exposure than noncontact sports, the greatest risk for the transmission of blood-borne diseases to or from athletes is during their off-the-field activities (Mast et al. 1995).

Due to the confidentiality of medical information and laws regarding disclosure of HIV status, HIV-infected athletes pose a potential threat to opponents. The current legal system in the United States has placed the responsibility for the sexual transmission of HIV with the HIV-infected person. However, no recorded cases of legal activity exist regarding who is responsible for the transmission of HIV during athletic competition. Participants in all sport activities, including the game officials, assume the risk of HIV transmission, just as they do for other injuries inherent to the sport in which they choose to participate. While the risks associated with participation in sport are not life threatening, the risks and mortality associated with HIV infection are well established (Mast et al. 1995; Seltzer 1993; Wolohan 1997; "The Medico-Legal Complexities of HIV and Athletic Competition" 1995). Until the courts are called upon to address the cause and effects of HIV infection via transmission during a sporting event, athletes and other game personnel infected with HIV will likely continue to participate while remaining silent about their disease.

Universal Precautions

Universal precautions, as described by the Occupational Safety and Health Administration (OSHA) guidelines, regulate the activities of many members of the athletic health care team (OSHA 1991; Ross and Young 1995). In 1992, the American Academy of Pediatrics (AAP), in their policy statement about HIV and sport, recommended the use of universal precautions adapted for the athletic setting (AAP Policy Statement 1992). Many athletic contests usually occur without any medical personnel in attendance. Therefore, one can reasonably anticipate that OSHA guidelines may be extended to include reasonable and prudent actions by coaches and officials determined to act as caregivers in these environments (Herbert 1993; Pollard and Godwin 1993). In fact, the position statement issued in 1995 by the American Orthopedic Society for Sports Medicine (AOSSM) and the American Academy of Sports Medicine (AASM) remarks, "All personnel involved with sports should be trained in basic first-aid and infection control." (AOSSM and the AASM 1995).

In any sporting event, game officials are charged with recognizing when an open wound presents an unacceptable risk to participants. Because any athlete may be HIV positive, prompt recognition and proper handling of bloody injuries and blood spills are essential. Universal precautions no longer deal exclusively with occupational exposure control plans but are becoming the community standard in the fight against the transmission of HIV. Everyone who has responsibility for user safety should give universal precautions the highest policy and operational priority (McAvoy and Dustin 1990). The sport arena is no exception. Additionally, because rules of competition have been modified to include methods of handling bleeding athletes and blood spills, game personnel may be held to a higher standard than previously experienced.

While the rules governing play are unique to each sport and, in many instances, each league, every organization that sanctions, supervises, or conducts sport events should have a statement of policy and procedures regarding the handling of a bleeding player and blood spills. Every injury that results in damage to the skin increases the potential for transmission of infectious diseases. Procedures must be followed to eliminate or minimize exposure to infectious agents. Every profession has a responsibility toward the persons who deliver their goods and services. These individuals must be educated about HIV, its incidence, its transmission, and its prevention, particularly when they have a reasonable chance of being exposed to blood or blood spills. Because few sports have zero risk, game officials, at some time, will probably be exposed to a bleeding athlete and/or a blood spill (Calabrese et al. 1993).

Sanctioned Competition

Presently, for many legal and ethical reasons, mandatory HIV testing of athletes or other game personnel does not exist. In 1993, three major governing bodies of interscholastic and intercollegiate sports issued guidelines and rules regarding the handling of blood. The National Collegiate Athletic Association (NCAA) Executive Committee endorsed a statement developed by the Committee on Competitive Safeguards and Medical Aspects of Sports regarding bleeding during practice or competition (NCAA 1993). The National Association of Intercollegiate Athletics (NAIA) included in their *Standard Operating Procedures for National Tournaments* basic guidelines for medical personnel concerning the handling of potentially infectious materials (NAIA 1993). In the 1993–94 rule changes for many sports, the National Federation of State High School Associations (NFSHSA) included procedures for officials to follow when they see blood on a player or uniform (Federation Rule Changes for 1994 1994). Interscholastic rules initially dictated a five-minute time limit to control bleeding by a player but were modified to "a reasonable amount of time" to be determined by the game officials. Cleanup time for blood spills and exchange of "saturated uniforms" is at the discretion of the referee. Intercollegiate rules do not designate time limits for controlling bleeding or to clean blood spills.

Collision and contact sports environments put their participants at a greater risk of blood exposure than noncontact or individual sports. Amateur wrestling has, perhaps, the highest incidence of direct skin-to-skin contact than any other sport in the United States (Dick 1995). Amateur wrestling in the United States is governed by three sets of rules: NCAA, NFSHSA, and USA Wrestling. The NCAA has issued the most extensive guidelines and explicit rules pertaining to blood-borne pathogens and communicable skin infections. The literature and position statements currently available address issues surrounding HIV-infected persons and their participation in sport. Even with explicit rules designed to protect individual participants, disclosure of HIV infection and prevention of HIV transmission remains the individual's responsibility (Harding 1993; Mitten 1994; Wolohan, 1997).

All organizations sponsoring sport activities need to develop responsible policies and demonstrate practices consistent with established guidelines for the prevention of blood-borne diseases (Bitting, Trowbridge, and Costello 1996; DeJoy, Gershon, Murphy, and Wilson 1996). Although the stated rules and procedures vary among sports and organizations, the bottom line is prompt, prudent intervention by the persons charged with supervising practice and play and the providing of medical attention. These persons are currently described as primary caregivers (AOSSM and the AASM 1995).

The NCAA, NAIA, and NFSHSA are only a few examples of bodies that govern athletic competition. The rules adopted by these organizations were designed to take responsibility for managing open wounds, bleeding, and blood spills away from the game officials. Aside from sport-specific strategies for stopping play, the general duty of high school and college officials is to stop play when an athlete is bleeding or has a bloody uniform. When bleeding occurs, the athlete is removed from the game to be treated by medical personnel. The NCAA rules require officials to stop the contest when a player has any amount of blood on his or her uniform and to permit an athlete to return to play only when given approval by medical personnel. The NFSHSA specifically requires that officials should stop the game when a player has an excessive amount of blood on his or her uniform. Upon reentry of the player to the game, the officials are to assume proper procedures have been followed. Several proverbial questions follow interpretation of these rules:

1. Who or what defines medical personnel?
2. What is considered an excessive amount of blood?
3. Does assuming that proper procedure has been followed meet today's moral, ethical, and legal standards of care for handling blood?

Many other organizations sanction, supervise, and conduct athletic events. Likewise, these organizations are responsible for adopting a set of rules and providing for adequate enforcement of these rules regarding bleeding athletes and blood spills (Brown, Phillips, Brown, Knowlan, Castle, and Moyer 1994). Rules should assure not only fairness but, more importantly, the safety of the participants. Such responsibility ultimately lies with the persons conducting the game—the game officials.

In order to understand the role of coaches, team officers, and medical personnel, *Article 10—Medical Service,* as specified in the International Rule Book & Guide to Wrestling (USA Wrestling 1997), is included here.

As specified in Article 7 of the Rules defining the international competitor's license, each wrestler must undergo a medical examination in his own country three days before leaving for Championships, Cups and Games. The organizer of the competition in question is obliged to provide a medical service to help detect individuals using drugs, conduct medical examinations prior to the weigh-in and give medical assistance during the bouts. The medical service must also assist in detecting doping cases. The Medical Service, which is required to operate throughout the competition, is under the authority of the FILA doctor in charge. Before the competitors weigh-in, the doctors shall examine the athletes and evaluate their state of health. If a competitor is considered to be in poor health or in a condition that is dangerous to himself or to his opponent, he shall be excluded from participating in the competition. Throughout the competitions, and at any time, the Medical Service must be prepared to intervene in case of an accident, and to determine whether a wrestler is fit to continue the contest. Doctors from the participating teams are fully authorized to treat their injured members, but only the coach or team officer may be present while treatment is being administered by the doctor.

The *USA Modification Rules* (USA Wrestling 1997), differ from the rules of the Fédération Internationale des Luttes Associées (FILA)—the international governing body of wrestling. The U.S. rules address all levels of competition conducted and sanctioned by USA Wrestling. The first rule discusses not only HIV infection but hepatitis B virus (HBV) infection as well. The *Blood Rule* specifically states the following:

1. Athletes known to be infected with the HIV/HBV cannot compete in any USA Wrestling sanctioned event.
2. Health care attendants known to be infected with HIV cannot administer to bleeding athletes.
3. Anytime an athlete bleeds during a bout, the action shall be stopped immediately and first aid administered.
4. A bleeding athlete cannot compete unless the bleeding and spread of blood is effectively stopped. If the spread of blood to others cannot be effectively prevented to the satisfaction of the Chief Medical Officer and officials, then the athlete cannot compete further.
5. Time outs to stop bleeding or the spread of blood shall not be included in injury time. The cumulative time out to stop bleeding and the spread of blood shall not exceed five minutes.

Community Programs

Recreation departments, youth sports associations, independent leagues, and church leagues customarily rely on hired individuals or volunteers to assume the roles of game officials. The recreation department director, association director, and league supervisor must address several questions about how bleeding players and blood spills will be handled and by whom. Are certain persons designated to handle bleeding players and blood spills? Do the persons assigned responsibility for handling bleeding players possess knowledge about HIV, its transmission, and use of universal precautions? Are the necessary items to practice universal precautions, such as disposable gloves, readily available for use?

Commonly in most recreation leagues, few or no qualified medical personnel are available to manage bleeding athletes or blood spills (Ross and Young, 1995). In such an environment, someone must be charged with ensuring proper handling of open wounds and blood spills if the risk of HIV transmission is to be minimized. Aside from the scorekeeper and league coordinator, who may or may not be present on-site, the game officials are the people consistently responsible for conducting a contest start to finish. An official, if determined to be the supervisor of a game, has a "duty to care"—that person must take necessary action to provide a reasonable, safe environment (Merriman 1993). Therefore, game officials should be ready to respond to a situation involving a bleeding athlete, even if only to provide rubber gloves and appropriate instructions for the person(s) rendering assistance.

Universal precautions are precisely what the words imply: precautions that everyone should observe. Whether a coach, manager, player, parent, or official, everyone should be educated about HIV transmission and prevention. In 1996, the CDC noted that the prevalence and incidence of HIV infection in the United States had begun to decline (Holmberg 1996). However, one of the foremost health concerns in the United States and the world is the incidence of HIV in the younger population, who could have an increased exposure to HIV via sport participation. For persons participating in sports, such as soccer, where the majority of participants are foreign-born, the risk of infection is greater (Irwin, Ouvo, Schable, Weber, Janssen, and Ernst 1997).

Risk Management

The responsibilities and assumed risk associated with sport participation impact all individuals who are involved. Attitudes about the "warrior-athlete" who is bleeding have changed. That individual is no longer looked upon as a hero or a star but as a potential source of HIV infection (Johnson 1992).

With risk management being a hot topic in today's corporate and professional society, it is only a matter of time until those who organize and conduct recreational and competitive sports events feel the need to inform all persons involved with event management about universal precautions. From the volunteer coach to the registered game official, all persons responsible for conducting a contest should be educated about the need to handle blood in a prompt, careful manner to reduce the risk and prevent the transmission of blood-borne pathogens, particularly HIV. Most first aid courses include instruction in the use of universal precautions. Local health departments, hospitals, colleges, universities, certified athletic trainers, and team physicians are excellent resources for obtaining user-friendly instructions and instructional materials regarding the proper handling of blood.

The basic elements of the risk management process have been identified (Cotten 1993). These elements may be adapted and incorporated into the training of every game official with little additional time commitment on the part of the certifying or supervising organization and the official.

• Identifying the potential risk for exposure to blood. While the risk of HIV transmission during participation in sport activities is extremely low, the exposure to exogenous body fluids is high. Exogenous fluids are those produced on the surface of the body, such as sweat. Contact and collision sports have the greatest potential for persons to be exposed to another individual's sweat, saliva, and blood. Among these, blood is the only body fluid known to transmit HIV.

• Evaluating the risks associated with improper handling of blood. HIV is a type of retrovirus transmitted through sexual contact, by parenteral exposure to blood and blood components, via contamination of infected blood into open wounds or mucous membranes, and perinatally from an infected mother to her fetus or infant. In the United States, less than one million persons are estimated to be infected with HIV. Although HIV infection in the United States has begun to decline and no cases of HIV infection occurring via sport activity has been documented in the United States, sport participation in any capacity poses a potential risk for HIV transmission.

• Select the proper approaches to minimize the risk of HIV transmission. The relatively low risk of infection cited in the literature does not minimize the need for technical information, education of sport participants, and infection control in athletic settings. Preventing the transmission of blood-borne pathogens is an important and complex issue for all practitioners involved in caring for athletes. Because individuals, including athletes, are most likely to acquire HIV while participating in non-sport-related activities, efforts to educate persons who choose to participate in organized sport may contribute to minimizing the overall risk of transmission of blood-borne diseases.

• Implement operating procedures that include having specific protective equipment and supplies at every contest. Pre-event preparation and observation of universal precautions requires little expense when compared with the deleterious effects of HIV infection and AIDS. Necessary equipment includes a designated receptacle for soiled equipment or uniforms and, where appropriate, a container for disposal of needles, syringes, or scalpels. Supplies include latex or vinyl gloves, disinfectant bleach solution, antiseptic, occlusive dressings, and bandages. In some instances, protective eyewear may be beneficial. Preventive measures that focus on recognition and immediate treatment of bleeding should not be left to chance.

Conclusion and Recommendations

Colleges, universities, high schools, parks and recreation departments, independent and church leagues, and youth sports associations should require their game officials to be educated about HIV transmission and prevention (American Alliance for Health, Physical Education, Recreation and Dance [AAHPERD] 1995). Additionally, these officials should be formally introduced to universal precautions and equipped with basic supplies to handle a bleeding athlete and a blood spill properly and safely. Preventive education is the most effective weapon in the prevention of HIV transmission. This is an instance where an ounce of prevention is worth a pound of cure.

Reasonably, contest officials are the only involved persons who could prevent serious injury while the contest (for example, wrestling or boxing) is in progress. The game officials are charged with and hold the responsibility of recognizing the potential of serious, unacceptable risk to participants. In the heat of activity, universal precautions have little meaning until the injury occurs. Therefore, the officials must always be aware that their job description includes the prevention of injury by anticipation as well as by enforcing the rules to the letter of the sport.

Thus, game officials educated about HIV transmission and prevention are better equipped to assist in effectively preserving the health and life of each participant. In instances where injury results in bleeding, they are able to promote a safe environment by reducing the potential for exposure to blood-borne pathogens. Successful prevention of transmitting HIV infection is possible only when preparation meets opportunity.

References

American Academy of Pediatrics (AAP) Policy Statement. (1992). HIV and sports. *The Physician and Sportsmedicine, 20* (5), 189–91.

American Alliance for Health, Physical Education, Recreation and Dance. (1995). *HIV Prevention Education for Physical Educators, Coaches, and Athletic Trainers.* Reston, VA: American Alliance for Health, Physical Education, Recreation and Dance.

American Orthopedic Society for Sports Medicine (AOSSM) and the American Academy of Sports Medicine (AASM). (1995). Human immunodeficiency virus (HIV) and other bloodborne pathogens in sports: Joint position statement. *The American Journal of Sports Medicine, 23* (4), 510–15.

Bitting, L.A., Trowbridge, C.A., & Costello, L.E. (1996). A model for a policy on HIV/AIDS and athletics. *Journal of Athletic Training, 31* (4), 356–58.

Brown, L.S., Phillips, R.Y., Brown, C.L., Knowlan, D., Castle, L., & Moyer, J. (1994). HIV/AIDS policies and sports: The National Football League. *Medicine and Science in Sports and Exercise, 26* (4), 403–07.

Calabrese, L., Haupt, H., Hartman, L., & Strauss, R. (1993). HIV and sports: What is the risk? *The Physician and Sportsmedicine, 21* (6), 173–80.

Cotten, D.J. (1993). Risk management—a tool for reducing exposure to legal liability. *Journal of Physical Education, Recreation & Dance, 64* (2), 58–61.

DeJoy, D.M., Gershon, R.R., Murphy, L.R., & Wilson, M.G. (1996). A work-systems analysis of compliance with universal precautions among health care workers. *Health Education Quarterly, 23* (2), 159–74.

Dick, R.W. (1995). HIV transmission unlikely in practice or competition. *Wrestling USA, 30* (8), 11.

Federation rule changes for 1994. (1994). *Referee,* (April), 60–62.

Hamel, R. (1992). AIDS: Assessing the risk among athletes. *The Physician and Sportsmedicine, 20* (2), 139–46.

Harding, T. (1993). Consensus on non-discrimination in HIV policy. *The Lancet, 341* (8836), 24–26.

Herbert, D.L. (1993). Clubs and the rule on bloodborne pathogens. *Fitness Management, 9* (1), 38.

Holmberg, S.D. (1996). The estimated prevalence and incidence of HIV in 96 large U.S. metropolitan areas. *American Journal of Public Health, 86* (5), 642-654.

Irwin, K.L., Ouvo, I.N., Schable, C., Weber, J.T., Janssen, R., Ernst, J. (1997). Absence of HIV-2 infection in a U.S. population at high risk for infection. *AIDS Weekly Plus,* March 31, 28–29.

Johnson, R.J. (1992). HIV infection in athletes. *Postgraduate Medicine, 92* (7), 73–80.

Mast, E.E., Goodman, R.A., Bond, W.W., Tavero, S., & Drotman, D.P. (1995). Transmission of bloodborne pathogens during sports: risk and prevention. *Annals of Internal Medicine, 122* (4), 283–86.

McAvoy, L.E., & Dustin, D.L. (1990). The danger in safe recreation. *Journal of Physical Education, Recreation & Dance, 61* (4), 57–59.

Merriman, J. (1993). Supervision in sport and physical activity. *Journal of Physical Education, Recreation & Dance, 64* (2), 20–23.

Mitten, M.J. (1994). HIV-positive athletes: When medicine meets the law. *The Physician and Sportsmedicine, 22* (10), 63–64.

National Association of Intercollegiate Athletics (NAIA). (1993). NAIA Standard Operating Procedures Concerning the Handling of Potentially Infectious Materials in *NAIA National Tournament Handbook.* Kansas City, MO: National Association of Intercollegiate Athletics.

National Collegiate Athletic Association (NCAA) Committee on Competitive Safeguards and Medical Aspects of Sports. (1993). Bloodborne pathogens and intercollegiate athletics in *NCAA Sports Medicine Handbook.* Overland Park, KS: National Collegiate Athletic Association.

Occupational Safety and Health Administration (OSHA). (1991). Occupational exposure to bloodborne pathogens. *Federal Register, 56* (235), 64175–82.

Pollard, G.W., & Godwin, D. (1993). Bloodborne pathogens: Developing an exposure control plan for university lifeguards to meet OSHA standards. *National Aquatics Journal, 9* (2), 4–8.

Ross, C.M., & Young, S.J. (1995). Understanding the OSHA bloodborne pathogens standard and its impact upon recreational sports. *Journal of the National Intramural Recreational Sports Association, 19* (2), 12,14, 16–17.

Seltzer, D.G. (1993). Educating athletes on HIV disease and AIDS—the team physician's role. *The Physician and Sportsmedicine, 21* (1), 109–15.

The Medico-Legal Complexities of HIV and Athletic Competition. (1995). *Sports Medicine Digest, 17* (7), 10.

USA Wresting. *International Rule Book & Guide to Wrestling.* (1997). Colorado Springs, CO: USA Wrestling.

Wolohan, J.T. (1997). An ethical and legal dilemma: Participation in sports by HIV infected athletes. *Marquette Sports Law Journal, 7* (2), 373–97.

Selected Readings for HIV Prevention and Control Guidelines

Consult the following list for details about HIV prevention and control guidelines issued by various organizations. For sport health care providers and coaches, Terry Zeigler has developed a practical guide for managing blood-borne infections in sport.

American Academy of Pediatrics Policy Statement. (1992). HIV and sports. *The Physician and Sportsmedicine, 20* (5), 189–91.

American Alliance for Health, Physical Education, Recreation and Dance. (1995). HIV Prevention Education for Physical Educators, Coaches, and Athletic Trainers. Reston, VA: American Alliance for Health, Physical Education, Recreation and Dance.

American Medical Society for Sports Medicine and the American Academy of Sports Medicine. (1995). Human immunodeficiency virus (HIV) and other bloodborne pathogens in sports: Joint position statement. *The American Journal of Sports Medicine, 23* (4), 510–15.

Brown, L.S., Phillips, R.Y., Brown, C.L., Knowlan, C., Castle, L., & Moyer, J. (1994). HIV/AIDS policies and sports: The National Football League. *Medicine and Science in Sports and Exercise, 26* (4), 403–07.

National Association of Intercollegiate Athletics. (1993). *NAIA National Tournament Standard Operating Procedures Concerning the Handling of Potentially Infectious Materials.*

National Athletic Trainers Association. (1995). Bloodborne pathogens guidelines for athletic trainers. *Journal of Athletic Training. 30* (3), 203–04.

National Collegiate Athletic Association. (1993, Summer). Sports committees incorporate bloodborne pathogens statement into respective playing rules. *Sports Sciences, 1,* 4.

National Collegiate Athletic Association. (1993–1994). *NCAA Sports Medicine Handbook.* Overland Park, KS: National Collegiate Athletic Association.

National Safety Council. (1993). *Bloodborne Pathogens.* Boston, MA: Jones and Bartlett.

Occupational Safety and Health Administration. (1991). Occupational exposure to bloodborne pathogens. *Federal Register, 56* (235), 64175–82.

World Health Organization, in collaboration with the International Federation of Sports Medicine. (1989). *Consensus Statement from Consultation on AIDS and Sports.* Geneva, Switzerland: World Health Organization.

Zeigler, T. (1997). *Management of Bloodborne Infections in Sport: A Practical Guide for Sports Health Care Providers and Coaches.* Champaign, IL: Human Kinetics.

CHAPTER 5

Reconstructing Lives: The Voices of Athletes with HIV/AIDS

Keith Gilbert
Queensland University of Technology, Brisbane, Australia

Research studies regarding differing aspects of the relationship between culture and sport litter sport sociology literature. However, a closer inspection indicates that researchers have literally forgotten one of the most important aspects of sport culture—the athletes themselves. Certainly, quantitative investigations have occurred. Unfortunately, very few studies have specifically been oriented toward qualitative research that includes a detailed examination of athletes' lives. In fact, athletes could be considered a marginalized group within society and in the cultural context of sport. Consequently, a dearth and subsequent need for substantive qualitative research into the culture of athletes' lives exists. This chapter attempts to fill this void by presenting a study using the life history method (Goodson 1992b) and narration (Hatch & Wisniewski 1995) as two complimentary qualitative perspectives. These further assist the development of research into athletes' lives. More specifically, life history research provides a solid base for understanding athletes' fears and concerns regarding a myriad of issues, including HIV and AIDS. Goodson (1992a) remarked that life history research "seeks to understand and give voice to an occupational group that has been historically marginalized." Clandinin (1992) stated that narrative provides insights into discussions of "particular situations in the context of the study being undertaken." This chapter addresses the void in the literature regarding a marginalized group of individuals, athletes who are infected with HIV or have developed AIDS.

As a precursor to this research, one must understand that very little sociological research has studied athletes with HIV/AIDS. This is surprising since HIV/AIDS is one of the most important social problems facing sport in the 20th century. Previous research has included biographies dealing with individual elite athletes such as Magic Johnson, Greg Louganis, Arthur Ashe, Tommy Morrison (see *Living With HIV/AIDS: Voices of Sports Professionals*, Chapter 6), and Tom Waddell. However, no one has attempted to discover how nonelite athletes cope with their predicament. This chapter is concerned about the experiences of gay and heterosexual men with HIV/AIDS involved in sport. What problems do they experience with the gradual degeneration of their bodies? How do athletes cope with this degeneration and the problems caused by this infection? What role does exercise play in their lives? What is their morality and ethics concerning sport? This chapter traces the loss of confidence, self-esteem, and changing identities as the bodies of these athletes gradually break down. It also discusses the extraordinary lengths infected persons go through, the determination they possess to maintain fitness and health, as well as their strategies to cope with the disease. Thus, this chapter focuses on the micropolitics these athletes face in the everyday sporting environment.

Methodology

This chapter has been developed to promote the voices of athletes with HIV and AIDS who choose to continue playing sport and who are marginalized in society. It asks these athletes questions about others' perceptions and the issues regarding their disease. It addresses some of their concerns about the gay and heterosexual communities and their interactions with HIV-negative people.

The analysis presented in this chapter is derived from data gathered from 10 athletes over a period of eight weeks in a North American city. The research methodology consisted of interviews and a focus-group interview involving eight of the athletes. All interviews were audiotaped and transcribed. The taped interviews, which lasted for approximately 30–40 minutes, were analyzed by creating transcripts. The researchers used a grounded-theory approach, as highlighted by Glaser and Strauss (1967), to analyze the data. After rigorously examining the data, they formulated further questions to use in the focus-group session. These subsequent interviews were also audiotaped, transcribed, and analyzed. Finally, the researchers asked the participants follow-up questions over the telephone and gathered additional data. A description that links the athletes' responses with the available literature follows. This provides ideas about the nature of the athletes' lives and the influence HIV and AIDS have had on their physicality. The chapter analyzes the results of the study according to the following issues: playing against others, body breakdown, resentment and anger, as well as physical problems.

Playing Against Others

In a recent conversation with an athlete, Chris, who is HIV positive, the author was struck by the veracity of his comments regarding the notion of him competing against athletes who are not infected.

> I don't think that athletes should really be concerned about my health problems. In fact, I think that most athletes are so dumb about AIDS that it really wouldn't matter anyway. After all, the problems only occur when scared, pathetic people become paranoid about themselves contracting AIDS. Most of them know fuck all about their own bodies. Why should they be worried about mine? I am very careful about contact and take every possible precaution and that's why I play in the queer league. Its ironic because I didn't give a shit about protection beforehand—know what I mean, man.

This comment is interesting, and it concurs with what Wulf (1996) remarks, "According to the U.S. Centers for Disease Control, a basketball player's chance of contracting HIV from incidental touching is one in 85 million." Nevertheless, Chris' comments could be classified as inflammatory and thoughtless, especially in light of the return of Magic Johnson to the National Basketball Association (NBA) in 1992 after declaring that he had contracted HIV. Greg Louganis, another high-profile athlete with HIV, risked marginalization by his actions in the 1988 Olympics. However, he chose to keep his HIV status hidden from everyone other than his coach and a handful of close friends and family. Indeed, fear of contracting the disease was substantiated when the World Boxing Organization stripped Ruben "Hurricane" Polacio of his boxing title when it discovered that he was HIV positive (Sutcliffe and Freeland 1995). The Australian basketball team's captain—the spokesperson for several Australian Olympic team members—also voiced concerns and initially refused to play against Magic Johnson at the 1992 Olympic Games. One senior medical officer also came out in support of the Australian team by suggesting that the Australian Olympic Committee boycott their basketball game against the U.S. team and the HIV-infected Johnson (Sutcliffe and Freeland 1995). However, Wulf (1996) suggests that the following comment by Charles Barkley, at that time with the Phoenix Suns, was typical of the thoughts basketball players had regarding Magic Johnson: "It's not like we're going out to have unprotected sex with Magic on the floor. We're just going to play basketball." In a related situation, all the athletes interviewed by the researchers were very conscious that they could place others into dangerous situations. Therefore, these athletes are careful not to play sport if they have open sores or cuts. For instance, one of the interviewed athletes, William, said the following.

I am careful to extreme about playing basketball with other athletes even though I know that some of them who are my friends are HIV positive. I never play team sports if I have a sore on my arm or leg or for that matter anywhere on my body. I take care not to share water bottles, et cetera with noninfected athletes or anyone. It seems ridiculous really especially after Magic Johnson set the precedent in the NBA. I find it interesting that even though I play sport, much of the sports which I play to help me keep fit are individual sports. I used to play all team sports, but since my illness, I have preferred to avoid problems and exercise myself.

Quotes like this one indicate that the social functions of sport are not really available to HIV-positive athletes who principally use exercise to assist their fitness. Thus, HIV-positive athletes become marginalized and unable to enjoy the normal pleasures of sporting groups. This feeling of marginalization was not experienced only by William; others, like Mark, described the loneliness of their lives.

It is very obvious that because I have HIV that people are going to be reluctant to play sports with me. Most of my friends who played pickup basketball still play but without me. One ex-friend told me to f—— off. After that, I decided to move interstate where I could go underground for a while. Being shunned by society sucks, but losing close friends is worse.

Loss of social contact is a major problem HIV-positive athletes face because most of them were gregarious and easily adapted to the sporting social scene in their local neighborhoods. One athlete compared the problem of marginalization to race by announcing,

> Now I have the worst of both worlds. I have AIDS and I'm black. I didn't have a chance in life. When I first contracted AIDS, I became a recluse and my fitness levels decreased. But now I have learned to live with it and have begun to play sport.

Anxiety and concern about what other people might think of them slowed these HIV-positive athletes' return to sport. In all but one case, when first diagnosed, the athletes stopped playing sport on doctors' orders or because they became so devastated by the news. All athletes found that playing sport gave them confidence and allowed them some enjoyment. As Roy commented, "It helped give me peace of mind because, initially, the burden of guilt was too much to endure." Sport then gives the athletes an opportunity to have renewed vigor and take charge of some of the life they are losing. Sport, therefore, appears to have a cathartic effect on athletes with AIDS, giving them some form of societal interaction with individuals who would be wary and mistrustful of them in any other scenario.

As Seltzer (1993) remarked, "Since the mid-1980s the HIV virus and AIDS has created an uncertain fear in the athletic arena." This was nowhere more obvious than when Magic Johnson attempted to return to the NBA prior to the 1992–93 season. Indeed, at this time, several prominent players expressed reservations about sharing the court with him (Reuters Information Services 1996). Vernon Maxwell of the Philadelphia 76ers commented about playing against an athlete with AIDS, "You get scratched on your hand and he might get an open wound. I don't want to be there with that. I have a wife and kids" (Wulf 1996). During his attempt to return to the NBA, many expressed uncertainty about whether Johnson would infect another player with the virus. However, since that time, concerns regarding the virus and sport appear to have decreased due to educational efforts. In fact, as Ken Rosenthal (1996) from the *Baltimore Sun* described, the press hailed Johnson's return.

> "Magic" Johnson is back and the world is a better place. It is better now because we know so much about HIV. And it's better because of the idea of Johnson playing basketball again, four years after he tested positive for the virus that causes AIDS.

The basketball players themselves were pleased to see Magic Johnson return to the game. For example, Michael Jordan noted, "I think it truly shows his love for the game, I wish him well." Charles Barkley of the Phoenix Suns referred to Johnson's comeback by commenting, "I wish him the best. I'm glad to see 'Magic' back on court." Apparently, at the elite level, players who are HIV positive can feel accepted. Yet, at lower athletic levels, the athletes rarely come out and state openly that they are HIV positive. Instead, they take their own precautions against infecting others. Playing with others then takes on a new twist.

Body Breakdown

Traditionally, the body and the mind have been treated as two separate entities–with greater emphasis on the mind. Thus, the centrality of the body to human life is not usually referred to from the perspective of "the homosexual". This is indeed surprising as the respondents in this study constantly referred to the concept of the body as an erotic image that directs their discourses about life. As Hall (1993) reminds us, "Homosexuality expresses something—some aspect of desire—which appears nowhere else, and that something is not merely the accomplishment of the sexual act with a person of the same sex."

That something—voyeurism—is also one of the most persuasive features of a person's bodily experience. The perceptions of the athletes' bodies and the relationship between desire and their disease were an important aspect in this study's findings. When elaborating on the problems he encountered, Bill explained that he was having serious difficulty coping with the breakdown of his immune system. He felt concerned that HIV was transforming him into a person different from the one he once knew.

> There is no doubt that my body has changed from a situation where I was fit, strong, and healthy to one where I can barely stand to look at myself in the mirror each morning. You know what I mean man? I was cut, chiseled, and really fine. You know those guys would comment on my looks and say, "Man you're the finest." You know what I'm saying? But I just can't work out like that no more. Those days are gone, man. Those days are gone. Long gone. I'm just different now.

In contrast, Robert and others interviewed felt that in the early stages, they had managed to maintain their previous fitness level and, more importantly, body shape and looks. These athletes accepted that at some stage, they might get sick. However, they were also cognizant of the role of fitness in their lives and the fact that they still wished to remain attractive to other men and wear smart clothes. Because of these reasons, most of the athletes worked out with weights every day as part of their routine. Most of them frequented local gymnasiums on a regular basis. They were, however, cognizant of the potential risk factors for others and took special precautions to avoid physical contact. Sam explained this as follows.

> Initially, I felt really sorry for myself, but after a while, I decided that I would live my life, one day at a time, and live my life to the full. Bodybuilding was my sport, and I still work out. Everyday I go to the gym and push weights with my friends although some days lately I feel weak and take it easier. My friends ask me what the problem is. I think they know but they don't say anything. But I know my shape is changing slowly, and I'm not sure how long I will be able to go to the gym. I really need the exercise because it has been part of my life for so long. I guess it's just another thing which I have to give up and come to terms with.

In many ways, the athletes have difficulties coping with the breakdown of their bodies because, according to Ralph, "There is a culture of the body beautiful among the homosexual population, which is part of the scene." The parading of the body in Gay Mardi Gras and maintaining a healthy image is all part of the culture of the gay athlete. As Waddell, a gay Olympian, remarked about fitness, "Exercise has always been my form of meditation. I draw great strength from it, physically as well as emotionally and intellectually" (Waddell and Schaap 1996). Indeed, *Los Angeles Times* reporter Robert Scheer (1996) referred to Waddell and his body in the following way:

> Dr. Tom Waddell, a tall, muscular, blond, Greek-god type when he represented his country in the 1968 Mexico City Olympics, still looks pretty good. Lankier now and bearded, in his favorite dress sweats and sneakers, he still suggests the supple strengths of the man who was once the world's sixth-best decathlon competitor. Not bad for a guy pushing 50. Not bad for someone dying of AIDS.

It is interesting that Scheer referred to Waddell's body in such a manner because the athletes in this study also worshipped their bodies. In fact, possessing a strong athletic body is an important part of their life, which they utilize to display their sexuality. To most of the athletes, their bodies are temples that they look after with great care. Sport gives them the opportunity to display their bodies in the societal context. As highlighted by Alan's comments, problems regarding the breakdown of the athletes' bodies and problems with their health are highly interrelated. For example, after hospitalization, the athletes would attempt to resume their regular fitness routines and play sport at the same level as before they became ill.

One athlete in the later stages of AIDS was unable to go outdoors to exercise because of embarrassing facial sores. Thus, he exercised each day at home for one hour. However, he found that the exercise exaggerated the problem and was forced to stop training. Sadly, it appears as though society cannot accept athletes with AIDS, and only a few organizations cater to HIV-positive athletes. The gradual breakdown of the health of the individual and the corresponding breakdown in his or her physique and physical capabilities must be addressed. All of the athletes considered exercise as a fundamental right and felt that it was an important parameter to maintaining their health and self-esteem. Chris explained these feelings by stating the following:

> If I can get out and run, I feel so much better. Um, it's as if I get a release of all the tension inside of me, and I feel free and invincible just like when I was a child. No one knows that I have a problem, and I can quickly run past people and greet them in a normal way. Last week, I ran with a friend who I overtook, and we chatted for about 20 minutes. It was great. I don't get the opportunity to do that in normal life. It's just one round of pills after the other, one round of checks after the other, and loneliness. Sport breaks the routine of waiting to die.

These words are very powerful. They highlight the plight of athletes who are not only marginalized in society but frightened by the gradual breakdown of their bodies. As a group, they were very concerned about their bodies and cognizant about their ability to function at a particular level. However, they were unsure of the manner in which their bodies will eventually break down. They were very tense about their appearance and what others thought of them. In general, these athletes would buy baggy clothes that hid particular individual problems. They were careful not to overtrain and worked out enough to maintain shape and form. Yet, they competed less and less as their illness progressed. Preferring to work out alone or with their partners rather than in the public domain increased their marginality and decreased their ability to cope with simple situations like taking public transportation to the clinic. Where possible, Mark and Bill, who were in the later stages of the illness, took cabs or drove themselves. However, few of the athletes went to public places. By comparison, in the early stages, they were more outgoing and expressed a positive body image. As Bill mentioned, "Sport really helped me feel like I was a normal person in a normal body." This feeling of self-worth is very important to HIV-positive men. The research by Sandstrom (1996) points directly to this fact. When referring to individuals with HIV, he commented:

> They often develop clearly visible symptoms of sickness, such as a pale complexion, an emaciated appearance, facial or bodily rashes, cancerous (Kaposi's sarcoma) lesions, or severe physical weakness. . . . This made it difficult or impossible for them to maintain the type of body appearance necessary to sustain conceptions of themselves as sexually desirable persons.

Rick, one of the participants in this study, poignantly stated the following:

> I can't really do exercises anymore for two reasons: one is that I have a port, the other is because of my loss of vision. I have a port because I have a catheter, and you have to be careful so the catheter doesn't separate. So body exercises are pretty much out of the question. And because of my lack of vision, I can't really go running. The only real option is to go swimming, and even that is a problem because the needle for the port is in five days a week and I can't swim when its in. So I really feel out of shape, you know. And that lowers my self-image. . . . I mean, I'm not a particularly vain person, but I used to have a nice butt and its gone. I just don't fill out my pants anymore.

In addition, Sandstrom (1996) found that when discussing how AIDS-related symptoms had affected an athlete's body image, one of his subjects, Matt, commented,

> I don't like my body anymore. . . . I used to feel good in it—now I don't. I don't really like the way it looks. I mean, all the KS [Kaposi's sarcoma] lesions—they're all over my body now. That doesn't make me feel very attractive.

This study recorded similar comments. For example, Ralph mentioned that he was uncomfortable with his physical appearance. He was highly critical of society when trying to come to terms with his sense of loss. He blamed society's lack of understanding for many of his own fears and frustrations. "I cannot go outside for fear of people's gaze," and "Society has to understand that we are not the modern-day lepers." On the other hand, Sam was much more interested in himself and his dual problems of body image and self-worth.

> My body is disgusting and totally fucked. It used to be so tight and muscular, but even after training, it's floppy. I am so self-conscious about the way I look and so sad sometimes about what I've lost. Sometimes I wish it were all over.

In summary, athletes appear to have several serious problems when they have to learn to cope with HIV/AIDS. These problems are mainly related to their physical appearance and loss of self-esteem. These individuals are concerned about the image they portray in their homosexual community and in society at large. Issues dealing with the visual impact of their disease seem to override any benefits that they might get physically and mentally from exercise. The athletes also experienced other difficulties such as the changed relationship with their bodies. They monitored everyday changes, which became the single most important focus in their lives. Whereas the notion of looking good used to be important, athletes with AIDS prefer to do the right things to make themselves feel good. They were, however, reluctant to give up exercise altogether and preferred to use exercise of some type to boost their often flagging spirits. The notion of the body as a symbol of good health and the associated benefits is something the HIV-positive athletes will never experience again. HIV appears to prey on their bodies and minds, causing them to hide from the rest of the community.

Resentment and Anger

From the beginning of this study, the athletes obviously felt angry and resentful about the problems they have encountered after contracting HIV/AIDS. These problems include resentment of healthy athletes against whom they were competing. This resentment occurred after games and during gym sessions where the HIV-positive athletes were overtly or covertly competing against the HIV-negative athletes. Basically, the HIV-positive study participants hated losing and being defeated in games that, previous to their illness, they could have easily won. Lack of energy often caused their defeats. Don explained these feelings.

> I used to win every tennis game that I played in this league. Now I have dropped down three leagues and every game is a battle. As often as not, I lose against opponents which I would have defeated two years ago. This has been a major problem for me because I have always hated to lose. In fact, I really couldn't believe that I had contracted AIDS. I thought this really can't be happening, this really can't be happening. When I started losing, I realized that I was only going to get worse.

This scenario occurs quite commonly among the athletes. As a result of a negative attitude toward life, they had to come to terms with whoever they could trust. In most cases, the first person they confided in, after speaking with their family, was their coach. For instance, Martin remarked, "Really had no choice but to tell my coach. I was an elite athlete and spent hours with him everyday." Martin also felt more anger because he was a nationally rated junior football player who had the potential to earn a scholarship to college and to enter the professional ranks. His resentment was obvious. He had contracted AIDS through a blood transfusion in his early teens when recovering from dehydration in a local clinic. This dehydration had occurred during summer football training. He also resents having to take ganciclovir prophylactically for oral herpes. He commented, "I am constantly reminded of HIV each morning when I see the pill bottles. Yeah! I'm really angry about that." Another athlete, Rex, shared similar views.

> I am really resentful of other men of my age. They can run, jump, and swim and be involved in activities with others. I guess I have this deep resentment inside which I could have kicked out of my system if I did not have AIDS and tire so quickly. It's a sort of curse, which I wish would just go away.

As Sandstrom (1996) remarked, "Disclosure of one's health status did not necessarily result in rejection" by other athletes, the coach, friends, or teammates. Most were sympathetic to the athlete's plight. However, some HIV-positive athletes experienced incidents and cases of rejection that certainly caused anger, resentment, and frustration. This primarily occurred because they became frustrated with their teammates' lack of knowledge regarding HIV/AIDS. Rex described this phenomenon quite strongly.

> I found myself getting very angry with my former teammates as they really disowned me, and it was terrible because we had won several junior college basketball games and championships together. Sudden rejection is something which all athletes need to know about. There should be some form of training program for all athletes so that they begin to understand the problems which can affect anyone of them at anytime.

In summary, as highlighted by the previous statements, resentment and anger is something that one needs to consider when working with HIV-positive athletes. At times during this study, the participants became angry about discussing their problems. For example, being shunned by society is very degrading for individuals who have always been naturally gregarious and outgoing. Coaches need to take this point into consideration and understand that they have a commitment to HIV-positive athletes over and above the regular call of duty. Indeed, coaches might be in a position to support HIV-positive athletes, who require some sensible outlet for their frustrations, fears, and pent-up energies. Sport, thus, could play an important role in their reeducation. It could allow these athletes to cope within a prejudiced society by aiding and supporting the reshaping of the athletes' social identities.

Physical Problems

All athletes in this study experienced physical problems. Most of them had difficulties with their medication. Many used the new type of drug called protease inhibitors, which controlled their viral replication. When tired, the athletes had lower viral replication rates and increased T-lymphocyte counts. This occurs when individuals are wasting (losing weight uncontrollably). Some of the athletes lost weight from their muscles and general body fat. This resulted in profound tiredness. The protease inhibitors assisted them to regain their immune capacity. Other athletes used a variety of drugs for a number of reasons. Unfortunately, either the drugs or the disease itself affected all of them at some time. They regularly became weak and lethargic. Interestingly, the sight of the former athletes now being weak and lethargic caused many of their friends to take up exercise and change their lifestyles. This occurred with Bill Toomey, an Olympic athlete who changed his lifestyle after meeting the HIV-infected athlete Tom Waddell in 1987. "The reunion had a profound impact on Bill Toomey. He stopped drinking that day, and went on a strict diet. Within six months he had shed thirty pounds, and he looked, and acted like an Olympic champion again" (Waddell and Schaap 1996).

Along with problems just described, the athletes faced other challenges such as coping with the sheer pressures of life. Their gradual physical breakdown some-times caused severe psychological problems that, in turn, led to lack of exercise and other physical traumas. Prior to the study, all the athletes could function well and play sport at a reasonable standard. However, after six months, some had experienced physical breakdown and yet others were unable to get to the interview sessions. In fact, it was very difficult to gather data due to the athletes' ongoing illness and the sensitivity of the task.

In summary, the athletes very carefully monitored their physical problems each day and were aware of any changes in their bodies. Some became psychologically disturbed and required extra drugs to combat the problems. Interestingly, their condition had profound effects upon other athletes and friends, some of whom changed their lifestyles significantly.

Conclusion and Recommendations

The previous data brought to the forefront the attitudes of HIV-positive athletes and the importance of sport as a vehicle to support the social construct of their lives. Clearly, more research needs to be attempted in this area because the marginalization of these athletes is of prime concern to them. This chapter highlighted the issues that HIV-positive athletes have to deal with on a daily basis. Their main concern was loss of social contacts that they had acquired through their involvement with sport. Their attitude toward others contracting the disease was admirable. Each athlete was genuinely concerned about the welfare of other athletes, whether they played on the same or on opposing teams. Thus, the athletes' caring attitudes specifically relates to them still wanting to be a part of society. Indeed, they craved acceptance and continually attempted to make amends for their social problems. The problems they encountered with the gradual breakdown of their bodies graphically highlights the sadness in their lives. Of interest here is the importance they placed on fitness and its relationship to self-worth. Their negative attitudes were understandable consid-ering their frustrations, anger, and remorse at the eventual loss of their physical abilities and loss of their attachment to sport.

A double-edged sword exists here. One edge activates protective mechanisms that force the athletes to fight discrimination and bias in the community, while the other is a point of uncertainty. Athletes competing with HIV know that they risk transmitting the virus to others. Thus, moral support and education for athletes without HIV/AIDS is essential because HIV disclosure, in essence, deprives individuals of the right to informed choice—potential victims also have rights. They have the right to accept or decline the risk. However, society has certainly arrived at a fused point of uncertainty involving a myriad of questionable issues that need further research. Until those issues are solved, caring, well-meaning, and informed coaches and trainers are needed to support HIV-positive athletes and educate athletes generally, because the ultimate risk is death.

References

Clandinin, D.J. (1992). *Classroom Practice: Teacher Images in Action.* London: Falmer Press.

Glaser, B.G., & Strauss, A.L. (1967). *The Discovery of Grounded Theory: Strategies for Qualitative Research.* Chicago: Aldine.

Goodson, I.F. (1992a). Exchanging gifts: Collaborative research and theories of context. *Analytic Teaching*, 15.

Goodson, I.F. (Ed.) (1992b). *Studying Teachers' Lives.* London: Routledge.

Hall, M. (1993). The male body in another frame: Thomas Eakins' the Swimming Hole as a Homoerotic Image. In *Journal of Philosophy and Visual Arts.* (1996). 8-22.

Hatch, J.A., & Wisniewski, R. (1995). *Life History and Narrative.* London: Falmer Press.

Reuters Information Services. (1996). *International basketball: Taiwan bars Magic.* Retrieved September 1, 1997 from the World Wide Web: **http://www.aImor53940HTM**

Rosenthal, K. (1996). Magic returns. *Baltimore Sun.*

Sandstrom, K.L. (1996). Redefining sex and intimacy: The sexual self images, outlooks, and relationships of gay men living with HIV/AIDS. *Symbolic Interaction. 19* (3) 241–62.

Scheer, R. (1996). Basketball report. *L.A. Times.*

Seltzer, D. (1993). Educating athletes on HIV disease and AIDS. *The Physician and Sports Medicine. 12*, 109–15.

Sutcliffe, M.A., & Freeland, D.K. (1995). Limits in confidentiality testing and disclosure with HIV infected sports participants engaging in contact sports: Legal and ethical implications. *Journal of Sport and Social Issues,* November, 415–31.

Waddell, T., & Schaap, D. (1996). *Gay Olympian: The Life and Death of Dr. Tom Waddell.* New York: Knopf.

Wulf, A. (1996). Sport and body science. In Callen, A. *The Spectacular Body: Science and Technique in the Work of Degas.* London and New Haven.

CHAPTER 6

Living With HIV/AIDS: The Voices of Sports Professionals

Deborah L. Keyser
Radnor School District, Pennsylvania

Arthur Ashe, Greg Louganis, Earvin "Magic" Johnson, Tommy Morrison—all were elite athletes in their respective sports. Despite other commonalities among the four, one specific circumstance is painfully apparent. All four have been diagnosed with the human immunodeficiency virus (HIV), which progresses to acquired immuno-deficiency syndrome (AIDS). Unfortunately, the stigmas and ultimate fatality that accompany this disease make it easier to call to mind their medical status than to remember their athletic accomplishments. Winning Wimbledon, four gold medals in the Olympic Games, five NBA championships, and a World Boxing Organization title are no match for the hype that an HIV-positive status can bring to a well-known public athlete. This chapter will examine the lives of four outstanding sports professionals, focusing on how they contracted HIV and how they dealt with its consequences. This chapter portrays their courage in the face of adversity, such as facing discrimination and loss of privacy. It also describes their strategies to overcome the physical, emotional, and social impacts of the disease.

Arthur Ashe

Arthur Ashe, the first African American tennis player to win Wimbledon, had a life filled with medical problems. His sickly childhood was a precursor of what his future would hold. Quadruple-bypass surgery in December of 1979 initiated Ashe's ongoing trips to various kinds of medical experts. On June 21, 1983, Ashe underwent a second heart surgery, this time a double bypass. The reentry into his sternum was more difficult the second time, leaving Ashe feeling worse than after the initial heart surgery. His doctor suggested transfusing two units of blood, a simple remedy to help Ashe get back onto his feet a little faster. Without hesitation, Ashe agreed and received the transfusion, which helped greatly in the short term. Unbeknownst to the medical team, the hospital, or Ashe, the blood was tainted with HIV. Arthur Ashe was 40 years old.

At the time, Ashe was the captain of the Davis Cup team. He had long ceased to be an active competitor but kept tennis as an integral part of his life. Ashe conducted clinics and worked at country clubs to teach youngsters about the game of tennis. Therefore, when he was diagnosed with HIV in September of 1988, his decision regarding his involvement in tennis did not involve his competitive career. HIV did affect every aspect of Ashe's life at the time, though, both personal and professional.

While vacationing with his family, Ashe awoke one morning to find that his right hand would not function. Despite efforts to move his fingers, he was unable to accomplish this task. After returning home to his Manhattan apartment, Ashe drove to his "second home," New York Hospital, for an appointment he had made regarding his hand. After numerous tests, ending with exploratory brain surgery, the results revealed that Ashe had an opportunistic infection of the brain called toxoplasmosis, a common symptom of HIV-positive patients. Arthur Ashe was diagnosed as HIV positive.

Ashe's reaction was a tribute to his strong character. His initial response to the news consisted of three words: "Aha" and "That's that" (Ashe and Rampersad 1993). In his autobiography, *Days of Grace*, Ashe wrote that at no time did he feel nervous or scared about his diagnosis. His wife had supported him throughout his previous medical ailments. She sat at his side, holding his hand, as he received this most recent medical news. He felt that receiving contaminated blood was simply unlucky (Ashe and Rampersad 1993). Ashe's positive attitude and lasting determination to live with this disease were inspiring. At no time did he feel as if he were being punished for a wrongdoing somewhere in his life. AIDS was simply another hurdle that he would strive to overcome.

Arthur Ashe clearly described the way he contracted the disease. His reputation was extremely important to him. The public often assumes that HIV-positive individuals are homosexuals or intravenous drug users. Because a successful tennis career and drug abuse would not have mixed well, homosexuality appeared to be the only other explanation. Ashe reported that he had never cheated on his wife with anyone. He also stated that the homosexual lifestyle was not his style, reiterating many times that he was not gay. Nevertheless, many people thought that Ashe might have been gay. In an interview, Larry King asked Ashe whether he had had a homosexual experience, a question about which America wondered.

After contracting HIV, Ashe felt the need to know more about the homosexual lifestyle in order to educate children, whether homosexual or heterosexual, about the ways in which they could protect themselves from HIV. Ashe felt very strongly about sex education and the importance of making the best decisions possible concerning sexual behavior. He not only spoke to children of all ages but also donated money to children suffering from AIDS.

HIV brings feelings of depression and despair to most who receive news that the test came back positive. Initially, Ashe did not feel much despair and actually lost little sleep over his medical condition. He did, however, read articles about HIV and AIDS. These eventually stimulated anxiety, making him aware of the illnesses and premature death that awaited him. Despite the grim outlook, Ashe actively participated in his treatment. He kept informed about new medications and talked openly with the medical team about his options. His medications included AZT, Cleocin, Leucovorin, Daraprim, and didanosine, to name only a few. His approximately thirty pills a day cost $18,000 a year (Ashe and Rampersad 1993). Ashe took a good look at AIDS, found its weaknesses, drew on his strengths, and did battle with the disease every day, just as he would an opponent on the tennis court.

Upon hearing of his HIV status, Ashe did not rush to the closest reporter to disclose this most personal piece of information. After his diagnosis, he and his wife kept the news as quiet as possible, until eventually, they became aware that someone had found out. Interestingly, a friend of Ashe's, also a reporter for *USA Today*, heard word of Ashe's condition. During a telephone conversation, the friend asked Ashe to confirm a lead. That's when Ashe knew he had to go public. On April 8, 1992, Ashe made the formal announcement. He did blame *USA Today* for forcing him to reveal a part of his life he had tried to keep private. Although he felt relief in his outing, Ashe resented being put into a position that would have forced him to lie if asked about his HIV status. His announcement to the public was filled with emotion and with gratitude to the medical professionals who had kept his secret for so long.

The public's reaction to Ashe's statement was overwhelming. *USA Today* received hundreds of letters criticizing their decision to run the story about Arthur Ashe, pushing him unwillingly into the limelight. Many who responded by letter and phone were so outraged that they canceled their subscriptions and compared the article with those in grocery store tabloids. Certainly, the right of privacy versus the rights of the press surfaced as a major issue. Ashe was stunned at the response and appreciative of the public's support. He received numerous letters from the public. Many consisted of remedies for HIV, including herbal concoctions, religious messages, and magical potions. Although Ashe appreciated the recommendations, he stuck to the advice of his medical team.

Before Arthur Ashe's death from pneumonia on Saturday, February 6, 1993 at New York Hospital, he devoted much of his time to raising money and public awareness in the fight against AIDS. After his public announcement, Ashe formed the African American Foundation for the Defeat of AIDS. Since he created this foundation to increase international aid, 50% of the money generated was sent to foreign countries (Ashe and Rampersad 1993). A few months later, the Arthur Ashe Foundation was formed. A tennis exhibition featuring the major male and female players of the time, namely John McEnroe, Andre Agassi, Pete Sampras, Jim Courier, Martina Navratilova, Steffi Graf, Pam Shriver, and Arantxa Sànchez Vicario, celebrated the foundation's beginning. Both professional and amateur tennis players were generous with their time and other invaluable contributions to Ashe's cause.

Ashe was a man of great integrity before and during his fight with HIV. His only real fear involved whether he had infected his family. Both his wife and daughter have been repeatedly tested, and both are HIV negative. In spite of all the medical disabilities Ashe dealt with, he always considered himself blessed. He prayed to God and thanked Him for the gifts he had received, never asking to be cured of any ailment. His supportive family, expert medical team, and positive attitude helped Ashe live. Although AIDS beat Ashe in the end, he never gave up battling the most fierce and unpredictable competitor he had ever faced on or off the court.

Greg Louganis

Unlike Arthur Ashe, Greg Louganis's life involved a constant search for acceptance and affection. He was adopted at a young age and was the focus of hurtful teasing during his early school years. His dark skin and his keen interest in acrobatics and dance did nothing to help camouflage his differences from other young boys his age. The difficult times he encountered in the classroom stemmed from dyslexia, which was not diagnosed until he entered college. Name-calling, beatings, and placement into special classes only made Greg's life more troublesome.

At age 12, Greg attempted suicide. His failure only deepened his depression. Around the same time, Greg's body began to wear down due to the great stress he had put on his joints during gymnastic and acrobatic routines. Despite his great success and many accomplishments, Greg had to forsake that interest and pursue only diving. By age 16, Greg qualified for the 1976 Olympic trials in Montreal in the 10-meter platform and the 3-meter springboard.

Greg Louganis left Montreal with a silver medal in the 10-meter platform and his first encounter with true love. His love interest was a member of the Soviet team. Although the relationship did not outlast the Olympics, Greg's sexuality suddenly became clear to him. Unfortunately, the struggle to please himself, his coach, and his father on the diving board while hiding his new homosexual identity laid the groundwork for two more suicide attempts, both unsuccessful.

Greg became involved in a few gay relationships, none of which materialized into anything long-term. Despite feeling good about himself, Greg got involved in a violent relationship. Years after the relationship ended, this man—Kevin—informed Greg he had tested positive for HIV. The year was 1987. Greg tested positive in 1988.

In 1984, the Olympics were held in Los Angeles. Greg won gold medals in the 3-meter springboard and 10-meter platform. Around the same time, Greg began a relationship with a man whom he identified as Tom. Early in the relationship, Greg was raped by Tom, marking the beginning of Greg's battle to keep Tom satisfied. Tom and Greg never discussed AIDS or HIV. Greg did not see it as a threat since he considered his relationship with Tom monogamous and felt as if he had never been promiscuous.

Greg was unaware of Tom's true lifestyle. Tom was a male hustler. Unfortunately, Greg was ignorant of that until long after Tom had gained control of Greg's personal and professional life. Tom manipulated Greg so well that Greg had appointed Tom as his manager. In fact, Tom gained full control of Greg's earnings and business deals. Greg took years of abuse from Tom and received great support from his friends before he put an end to the relationship.

In 1987, Tom was diagnosed with shingles. Also during this same period, many of Tom's friends tested positive for HIV. Neither Greg nor Tom got tested, completely denying that they were both at risk. By 1988, Tom was having trouble breathing, suffering from night sweats and high fevers. The Olympics were five months away.

Ironically, Greg and Tom both got tested on the same day, unbeknownst to each other. Tom had developed PCP (*Pneumocystic carinii* pneumonia), a symptom of full-blown AIDS. Not surprisingly, both tests came back positive. Greg was not sure whether this development would keep him from competing; the Olympics had no rules in place to deal with this situation. At that time, no other athletes competing in the Olympics had ever tested positive for HIV. Greg's emotions, especially anger, ran extremely high. He felt he had already overcome more in his life than most do in a lifetime. He also felt that he deserved to be HIV positive because of his sexuality.

Greg told few people and decided to keep training. He eventually had to inform his coach because of the medication's effect on his rigorous physical and mental workouts. Ron, his coach, was extremely supportive and tried to keep Greg from sinking deeper into depression. Somehow, Greg made it through the Olympic trials and began preparing for the preliminary events.

It was the ninth dive on the 3-meter springboard in the 1988 Olympics. Greg prepared as he always did before executing any dive. On this particular dive, however, Greg got too close and slammed his head onto the board, hitting the water with a thud. As he struggled out of the pool, holding the top of his head, Greg began to panic. He panicked not only about the scores he would receive for the dive but about the HIV-positive blood dripping down the back of his neck. Greg could only hope that he had not bled in the pool. He also hoped that the doctor who stitched his head without wearing gloves or any personal protective equipment would not become infected. Greg was too scared to say anything to anyone about his condition, fearing he would be unable to continue in the competition. Somehow, some way, Greg returned to the springboard and later won a gold medal on the 10-meter platform.

After the Olympic Games and many interviews and appearances, Greg realized that Tom was taking full advantage of his successful diving career and doing nothing to enhance the relationship romantically. As Greg attempted to leave the relationship, Tom threatened to inform the public of Greg's homosexuality. Tom also threatened to go one step further by reporting that Greg had infected Tom with HIV. In the face of Greg's great fear of being outed as well as his feelings of loss about the ending of a long-term relationship, Tom agreed to a settlement in which he received much more than he deserved. Tom died not long after the end of the relationship in the home he had shared with Greg.

Greg announced his retirement at the conclusion of the 1988 Olympics. He used his time to rebuild the damaged relationship with his father. Since his father had become ill with cancer, they talked in depth about mortality. Greg informed his father about his sexuality and AIDS diagnosis. For once, Greg's father did not condemn him. The old wounds that had never healed for Greg finally closed by the time his father passed away. As those around Greg died, he began to fall again into a deep depression, awaiting his turn to face death.

Greg had to overcome adversity again. First, he had to shake an addiction to morphine and codeine. Then he contracted a fungus called intestinal histoplasmosis that eventually landed him in the hospital. His interest in acting, which he had pursued throughout his life, finally gave him the lift that he so desperately needed. Greg got the role of a gay man with AIDS in the play *Jeffrey*. At this point, it is a wonder that Greg's sexuality was still in question. How could the public not realize that Greg was gay? Apparently, according to Greg, the reporters realized and simply stopped asking questions.

After the play had ended and Greg overcame another addiction, this time to Percocet, he decided to write *Breaking the Surface*, an account of his life story. By writing about his life, leaving no stone unturned, Greg decided to announce his homosexuality and make it publicly known. Greg's outing came at the Gay Games IV in 1994. A video was played of Greg first diving and then announcing a welcome to all the athletes. He stated that it felt great to be "out and proud" (Louganis and Marcus 1996). Needless to say, all the gay athletes at the games cheered and applauded the announcement that, for Greg, was so painfully difficult.

Greg's accomplishments go well beyond the writing of his book. He played an instrumental part in moving the volleyball preliminaries for the next Olympic Games out of Cobb County, near Atlanta, where gays were openly not welcomed. Greg has also become involved in other AIDS organizations like PAWS (Pets Are Wonderful Support). This organization takes care of pets owned by AIDS patients as well as taking pets to visit AIDS patients.

Greg did interviews with Barbara Walters and Oprah Winfrey. He received tremendous public support for announcing his health concerns. He has adopted a great attitude about himself, which took many years and much therapy. Currently, he is continuing the fight against AIDS and getting involved in things that bring him joy. These include acting, teaching dance, showing his dogs, and dating. It is hard to believe that throughout Greg's successful years of diving, he carried with him so many serious issues.

Earvin "Magic" Johnson

The equivalent to Greg Louganis on the 10-meter platform is Earvin "Magic" Johnson on the basketball court. One of seven children, Earvin was raised in Lansing, Michigan. He grew up improving his basketball game on any court he could find. His hard work paid off as early as junior high school; Earvin had already surpassed the rest of the athletes at his school. Upon graduation from high school, Earvin entered a primarily white college, Michigan State University, that was just crossing the segregation barrier.

In 1978, Magic made the cover of *Sports Illustrated,* which featured an article about outstanding college sophomore basketball players. That same year, Michigan State University made it to the NCAA Final Four. Magic was facing Indiana State, which had a player of equal caliber, Larry Bird. Michigan State University won that game and also won the tournament title. At that point, Magic made a major life decision. He left Michigan State University after his second year to join the Los Angeles Lakers in the National Basketball Association (NBA). For more than 10 years, Magic Johnson was an elite point guard. He led his team to five NBA championships, two of them falling in consecutive years. He won the Most Valuable Player (MVP) award three times, demonstrating that Magic was a force and a legend on the court.

Although Magic is tremendously proud of his performance on the court, his past performance off the court has been his focus most recently. When Magic was attending Michigan State University, he dated plenty of women. He met one special woman, Cookie, who remained a part of Magic's life after college. The NBA lifestyle was also conducive to the lifestyle Magic had become accustomed to in college. Women were everywhere the Lakers went. Women waited outside the arenas, in hotel lobbies, at restaurants, at clubs, everywhere the team might be found. Because most of the players had wives and girlfriends, the players were very discreet. Magic, dating Cookie off and on throughout this period, never became emotionally involved, and he never let a woman stay overnight in his hotel room. Of course, this was not merely to protect Cookie. It mostly had to do with his performance on the basketball court. Magic made it clear to everyone, Cookie included, that basketball came first.

Cookie was not unaware of Magic's lifestyle. Despite urging from her friends and family to discontinue the relationship due to Magic's lack of commitment, Cookie held on. She knew that Magic loved her. However, she also understood his attitude about basketball as well as the opportunities available to him because of his star status. After two broken engagements, Cookie and Magic finally walked down the aisle on September 14, 1991. It was the happiest day of Magic's life.

During his years of sexual promiscuity, Magic never considered the threat of HIV. As most do, he thought that since he was not gay and did not use intravenous drugs, he was not at risk. Just prior to a preseason exhibition game in 1991 versus the Utah Jazz in Salt Lake City, Magic received a call from the team physician saying he had failed the insurance physical exam and needed to return home immediately. Magic was on the next plane to Los Angeles, nervous about the news but unable to identify what could possibly be the matter.

On Friday, October 25, 1991, Magic received the news from the doctor that his blood tested positive for HIV. He was in complete shock. Magic was not sure how this would affect his career but more importantly, how would his wife react? He and Cookie had been keeping secret that she was pregnant. What would be the baby's condition? Magic returned home immediately to inform Cookie about his health.

Cookie was devastated that Magic had tested positive for HIV. She and the baby were both tested soon after hearing the news. Magic was retested with a more accurate assay to confirm the information. Magic came up positive. Cookie, and therefore the baby, both tested negative.

Magic's fellow competitors urged him to retire. The season began with Magic sitting out, claiming to suffer from the flu. No other professional athlete who was still active in his or her sport had ever been diagnosed as HIV positive. No precedent had been established. Magic decided to retire and did so by announcing his HIV status at a press conference on November 7, 1991.

Like Arthur Ashe and Greg Louganis, Magic became an activist in the fight against AIDS. He also received bushels of letters that contained medicines and remedies to cure AIDS. Yet, he did what Ashe and Louganis did. He began taking AZT and other drugs. Magic also learned as much as possible about the disease and gained a better understanding of those who suffered from it.

Soon after his announcement, Magic received a letter from President Bush, asking him to join the National Commission on AIDS. Magic did join. Magic met with President Bush, who encouraged him to play a more influential role in the fight against AIDS. Magic did what he could on the commission. Not long after accepting the position, Magic wrote a letter to President Bush stating his disappointment with the President for not leading the charge against AIDS and resigned. He did not feel as if the President was doing enough with the commission's findings to help the cause. Magic decided to continue on his own and do the most that he could with the help of those around him.

Magic did a few interviews soon after his announcement, one in particular with his friend Arsenio Hall. Arsenio asked Magic a pointed question about his sexuality, about which all of America was curious. How did Magic contract the disease? Arsenio asked Magic the question, and Magic responded that he was not gay. The audience applauded. Their applause confused Magic and infuriated the gay community. The applause signified that even though an individual had HIV, as long as the person was not gay, he or she would not be ostracized. At the time, Magic did not understand the issue. After the interview, Magic made an effort to understand the gay lifestyle.

Magic also educated the public by writing a book. He wrote *What You Can Do to Avoid AIDS.* It was aimed at young people and used vocabulary they would understand. Unfortunately, some bookstores found the book too explicit and would not put it onto their shelves.

The NBA and Nestlé teamed up to sponsor Magic in a Nickelodeon show called *A Conversation with Magic Johnson.* Youngsters could ask Magic questions concerning HIV and AIDS. He also formed the Magic Johnson Foundation to help raise funds for AIDS research and education. Like Ashe and Louganis, Magic Johnson became very involved in the fight against HIV and AIDS.

On February 9, 1992, Magic played in the NBA All-Star Game. Both teams were very supportive, and the crowd was ecstatic. Magic was still in training for the 1992 Olympics in Barcelona, so he had not fallen out of shape. One week after the All-Star Game, the Lakers retired Magic's jersey during the halftime of a Lakers-Celtics game. Magic, still high from the excitement and accomplishments in the All-Star Game, did not really want to retire. He felt healthy. Receiving the MVP award following the All-Star Game proved he could still compete with the best. A few weeks prior to the start of the following season and after the Dream Team's triumph at the Olympics in 1992, Magic announced his return to regular-season play.

Magic's return went as planned. HIV was just another challenge he had to meet on a daily basis. Unfortunately, soon after his return, a small cut on his arm during a game struck fear into the hearts of his peers. On November 2, 1992, Magic retired again, concerned that the fear he aroused in his opponents was not due to his skill but to the virus in his blood. Magic did not feel angry at the players who objected to his playing. He felt disappointed that they had not come to him first to ask questions and get some informed answers.

Magic's other fear stemmed from his retirement in November. While feeling obligated to leave the league due to his HIV status, he felt that other players in the league who pursued a lifestyle similar to his, and were therefore at risk, might resist getting tested. If retirement resulted from a positive HIV test, who would volunteer to be tested? Magic's fear may have become a reality since no other players have publicly announced their testing.

Four years later, in 1996, Magic once again returned to the NBA. Teams, coaches, trainers, and equipment managers had all been educated about HIV and AIDS. Everyone who came into contact with any bodily fluids used universal precautions to ensure that no harm would come to any individual. Magic felt the time was right to return to professional basketball. He did not have too many words for those who still opposed his return. Those who had been educated about HIV knew they had an extremely remote chance of becoming infected on the basketball court.

Yet, what if the situation had been different? What if Magic had contracted the disease through a homosexual encounter? What if Magic Johnson, a hero to every player and fan, did not contract HIV but, instead, a mediocre player who was not as well-known had contracted the virus? Would that person have gotten another chance or two? Would he or she be welcomed? Would the opposing words of teammates be hushed?

Tommy Morrison

Tommy Morrison's lifestyle paralleled that of Magic Johnson. Although Magic's fame stemmed from his performance on the basketball court while Tommy's fame originated in the boxing ring, both athletes found themselves in a position where women were constantly available. Tommy tested positive for HIV in 1996.

Tommy Morrison grew up in Jay, Oklahoma. His hard-nosed personality led him to enter toughman competitions at the young age of thirteen. Tommy's mother, Diana, convinced Tommy to bypass a college education and join the Kansas City Golden Gloves in 1988. Tommy did well enough to turn professional. Only a few years later, Tommy's success escalated to a 28 and 0 record, 24 of the victories from knockouts. A role in *Rocky V,* a Sylvester Stalone movie about a boxer, contributed to Tommy's success at the time.

Tommy enjoyed the highlight of his boxing career in 1993 and overcame his 1991 knockout loss to Ray Mercer when he defeated George Foreman for the World Boxing Organization (WBO) title. Unfortunately, the belt did not last long around Tommy's waist because Michael Bentt beat him and took the title.

In spite of Tommy's boxing record, his boxing career offered limited celebrity status until Don King entered the picture. Don King, the infamous boxing promoter, grabbed hold of Tommy's future after a loss to Lennox Lewis in October of 1995. He put Tommy to work and scheduled him to fight Arthur Weathers on February 10 and other opponents in March. These fights lead to a culminating bout with the legendary Mike Tyson.

Before the bout, Tommy Morrison was given an HIV test, a mandatory action before a boxing match in Nevada. The bout was canceled when the test came back positive. A few days later, after a second test confirmed his HIV status, Tommy appeared at a press conference in a Tulsa hotel to inform the world that he had been diagnosed as HIV positive.

Tommy, like Magic, led a promiscuous life. Especially after his acting debut, Tommy had no trouble finding a willing partner and described women as "expendable" (Hoffer 1996). He knew about safe sex but never practiced it. The public in general, Magic Johnson, and Tommy Morrison commonly thought that only intravenous drug users and homosexuals contracted HIV. Unfortunately for Tommy, he learned the lesson too late.

Tommy Morrison had been previously tested for HIV—with negative results. Three years before, some U.S. boxing commissions did require testing before bouts. Today, Georgia, Arizona, Washington, Nevada, New Mexico, Oregon, Utah, and Puerto Rico require HIV testing for boxers. Certainly the privacy issue continues to be a topic for debate. However as boxers continue to test positive, many other U.S. boxing commissions may consider mandatory testing. So far, seven boxers, including Tommy, have tested positive. Boxing is a bloody sport; the risk of infection is more of a threat during a boxing match than during a basketball game. No one disagrees with that.

Tommy's major concern was not his health but the health of women he may have put into jeopardy. Tommy had asked his high school sweetheart to marry him, and she accepted just after he defeated George Foreman. It seemed as if Tommy were turning his life around. Yet, the discovery of his HIV status transformed Tommy even more into a person who regretted his past and dreaded the consequences that others would have to suffer due to his irresponsibility. Tommy's fiancée tested negative.

Tommy contacted Magic Johnson, who convinced Tommy to join the fight to beat AIDS. Tommy is doing his part by speaking at high schools and colleges, encouraging students to do what he did not—practice safe sex. Yet the reaction to Tommy's announcement, at least in his hometown of Jay, Oklahoma, was mixed. A few weeks after his news became public, a sign proclaiming Jay the home of Tommy Morrison was taken down. Obviously, his promiscuity and HIV status did not elicit sympathy from all Americans.

Conclusion and Recommendations

Tommy Morrison, Greg Louganis, and Magic Johnson remain healthy despite their HIV status. Their lack of symptoms and ill effects from the disease send many mixed messages to athletes as well as to the public. Since these men generally appear to be healthy, the seriousness of the disease may not be apparent to everyone, especially young people. Furthermore, because not everyone who suffers from HIV or AIDS has the resources and support that these three athletes have, the battle against HIV may seem much more difficult for those lacking the financial resources to fight the disease. Finally, on a positive note, Tommy, Greg, and Magic offer a glimmer of hope by their ability to hold the disease at bay.

Whether someone contracts HIV through a blood transfusion, homosexual activity, or heterosexual activity, HIV has disastrous effects. How a person contracts HIV should make no difference; AIDS is not a form of punishment. For that reason, all athletes (professionals and nonprofessionals) living with AIDS deserve the same support, encouragement, medical care, and resources to fight back. Magic, Tommy, and Greg are fighting along with thousands of other athletes whose stories will never appear in print or be told.

References

Ashe, A., & Rampersad, A. (1993). *Days of Grace*. New York: Knopf.

Hoffer, R. (1996, February 26). I have never been so wrong in my life. *Sports Illustrated, 84*, 48–51.

Louganis, G., & Marcus, E. (1996). *Breaking the Surface*. New York: Plume Printing.

Selected Readings

Brown, C. (1996, January 30). Johnson is meeting less resistance. *The New York Times,* pp. B11, B13.

Eskenazi, G. (1996, February 16). Morrison speaks and proves full of remorse. *The New York Times,* pp. B7, B14.

Friend, T. (1996, January 30). After 4 years, his return begins tonight. *The New York Times,* pp. B11, B13.

Johnson, E., & Novak, W. (1992). *My Life.* New York: Random House.

McCallum, J., & Kennedy, K. (Eds.). (1996, February 19). Scorecard. *Sports Illustrated, 84,* 14.

Plummer, W., & Harmes, J. (1996, March 4). Sucker Punch—Tommy Morrison never knew what hit him: HIV. *People Weekly, 45,* 93–94.

Reilly, R. (1996, February 12). Welcome back! *Sports Illustrated, 84,* 22–31.

Smith, G. (1996, February 12). True lies. *Sports Illustrated, 84,* 32–42.

Vecsey, G. (1996, January 30). Magic plays for himself and others. *The New York Times,* p. B11.

Vecsey, G. (1996, February 16). Morrison didn't pay attention. *The New York Times,* p. B7.

CHAPTER 7

HIV and Sport: Constructing a Framework for Ethical Deliberation

Rodger L. Jackson
Richard Stockton College of New Jersey

Many of the difficult ethical problems that trouble people today in their deliberations about HIV were visible early in the spread of this virus. Even before AIDS had progressed from an obscure medical condition to the pandemic it is today, all signs indicated that it was not a simple, purely medical problem. Individuals quickly realized that the significant ethical issues associated with AIDS would not go away. Many first thought of this disease as having a mysterious origin and mode of transmission. It caused dreadful physical manifestations and early demise in social groups already marginalized in society—gay men, intravenous drug abusers, and individuals from foreign countries. Persons with HIV, their family and friends, health care workers, researchers, and policy makers all had to make important decisions concerning various aspects of this disease and its consequences. At times, these decisions had to be made relatively quickly with inadequate information. Sometimes grief, disgust, terror, or even hatred complicated the decision-making processes. Presumably, however, those making the decisions as well as those looking on wanted the decisions to be good ones. They wanted to take the right stands and to do the right things.

During the last several years, the medical community has learned a great deal about HIV and its modes of transmission, treatments, preventive measures, and the like. Other chapters in this book contain much of this information. Knowledge alone, however, does not resolve the complex ethical issues surrounding this disease. Knowing that certain behaviors put people at risk for HIV does not determine whether the public should require testing of individuals engaging in those behaviors. Contact with infected blood is one way to transmit HIV. However, knowing this does not decide whether HIV-positive individuals should be banned from activities where their blood may come into contact with others. Scientific knowledge alone cannot provide the answers to ethically problematic situations.

Ethics, as a branch of philosophy, is the discipline concerned with questions like the following. What is the right stand to take in a certain case? What is the right thing to do? What kind of person should I be? What sorts of goals and commitments should we as a society have? What are my obligations to others and to myself? When defined this way, ethics is clearly not so much about the way things are as it is about the way things ought to be. Making a decision that things are or are not as they ought to be is an extremely complex task. People cannot always achieve a consensus in ethically complex situations. The process of ethical inquiry, however, can lead to substantial results even if a final answer or the ultimate truth remains unattainable. These benefits include value clarification, reasoned justification for beliefs and actions, consistency and accountability for actions, and participation in the moral community. This process and its benefits will be more visible by examining questions in practical ethics.

When arguing a practical ethics question, individuals are typically debating a recommendation about how people ought to think or behave. This occurs whether they are discussing business, engineering, medicine, law, or HIV and sport. Such recommendations may be between two individuals or a policy governing many people. For instance, persons might be debating whether athletes have a moral obligation to inform their trainers of their HIV status or whether colleges ought to prohibit HIV-positive athletes from playing in contact sports. When considering such recommendations, individuals are not so concerned about the way people are behaving or thinking now or about what the law or institutional policy is now. Rather, individuals are concerned about whether they believe such recommendations ought to be. A proposal about how individuals ought to be conducting their lives, all things considered and regardless of the way things are now, is typically under consideration.

Conducting an exhaustive analysis of all possible ethical recommendations regarding HIV and sport is impossible. Many ethical issues are involved—mandatory testing, voluntary testing, banning of athletes, and personal obligations to teammates, for instance. Sport encompasses a diverse range of activities—tennis, basketball, football, diving, boxing, and figure skating, for example. Also, a wide range of professions are connected with sport—athletes, trainers, coaches, physicians, equipment handlers, college administrators, team owners, unions, and so on. The variety of ethical issues, the diverse range of activities covered under the general category of sport, and the wide range of professions connected with sport prevents exhaustive analysis here. It also cautions against making sweeping generalizations. The fact that ethics itself is filled with alternative theories and approaches further complicates this inquiry.

This variety and the complexity of ethical analysis is not unique, of course, to the area of HIV and sport. An intense ethical debate may strike some as akin to a melee out on the field. You are somehow in the middle of a whirling mass, maybe unsure how it started. When it is over, nobody seems to have won—although several may be considerably bruised. Seemingly, no rules, no goal lines, and no referees exist. This view, however understandable, can lead to some undesirable consequences. For example, some may simply accept an ethical stance without closely examining its justification or consequences. For instance, an individual may simply accept what family, friends, or colleagues advocate. Instead, an individual may endorse a view that any ethical stance is of equal worth—regardless of its justification, reasonableness, or merit.

Throwing our hands up and concluding that an analysis of the ethical issues surrounding HIV and sport is a fool's mission would be a mistake. All people have an important goal: to do the right thing. This goal may be particularly hard to reach when persons experience fear, ignorance, prejudice, or uncertainty. In order to reach the goal, to structure the ethical analysis, and to weed out inappropriate fears and prejudices, people need a framework that will guide them in their deliberations.

The next section of this chapter will outline a framework for ethical inquiry that takes into account the particular kinds of problems that arise regarding HIV and sport. Making this framework clear will be more useful to the readers than a more superficial exploration of several different ethical questions. However, just as reading about a sport is much different than seeing it in action or being a participant, just reading about an ethical framework is not enough. Individuals need to see how it can be used and then use it themselves. After presenting this framework, the author will then demonstrate its use by analyzing in some depth a specific ethical question regarding HIV and sport: Should HIV-positive boxers be prohibited from boxing?

Constructing a Framework for Ethical Deliberation

This section will first examine a discussion about a common topic in HIV and sport: whether college athletes ought to be tested for the virus. In a roundtable discussion sponsored by *Sports Medicine Update*, Len Hartman, a football player at Ohio State, made the following recommendation,

> I would like to see voluntary testing implemented. I would like to know how many of the people I line up against on Saturday afternoons are infected. . . . If I had to play against Magic Johnson, or a football equivalent of Magic Johnson, I don't know if I would be as aggressive. In fact, I would try to have the least amount of contact with that person as possible. That's detrimental to the game and that's detrimental to the sport in general. . . . Look at it from the athlete's perspective. Let's say, for instance, that you were in a fist fight, which is similar to playing football. Would knowing your opponent was HIV positive change the way you fought? . . . I've never played in a football game in which I did not bleed or have blood on my hands or arms. Even if you know that the risk of contracting the virus is small, it still affects the way you deal with that person. (Calabrese et al. 1993)

Specific Recommendations

With HIV and sport, the old adage that the devil is in the details is very true. Many have been in discussions where the arguments on both sides may be going nowhere and the frustration grows as the other side seems to miss the point. Then a third party listens to both sides and points out that the two actually agree with each other. However, they have been expressing identical positions in different language. If both sides had started by clearly stating exactly what they were proposing, they might have avoided the entire debate. Moreover, in committing themselves to such specificity, they also force themselves to reflect on what they are proposing and whether they truly believe it.

For example, take Mr. Hartman's recommendation to institute voluntary testing for anyone involved in a college- or university-organized sport. While the author has frequently heard students and colleagues debate this recommendation, it cannot be critically evaluated as it stands. Before examining a question of this sort, a number of items need to be specified. Would testing occur for all sports or only for contact sports? Would students with athletic scholarships lose them if they chose not to play after discovering themselves to be HIV positive? How would testing be financed? Would intramural sports be included or is the proposal restricted to intercollegiate sports? Would information about the HIV status of college athletes be gathered? Who would have access to this information? How would it be used? The point is not that making a recommendation is impossible because some further aspect will always need to be considered. Rather, the point is to recognize that terms like voluntary testing, banning from play, or informing the relevant parties can mean entirely different things depending upon how they are specified. Recommending an aggressive campaign of voluntarily testing intercollegiate athletes playing full-contact sports that includes contact tracing but no follow-up counseling significantly differs from recommending that universities supply athletes with home test kits. Both can be called voluntary testing, but they are hardly the same thing.

Expectations of the Recommendations

When Mr. Hartman recommended instituting voluntary testing, he did not do so because such testing is worthwhile in and of itself. Presumably, he recommended this to help achieve some goal. To evaluate the recommendation fully, readers need to know what the goal is. Unfortunately, Mr. Hartman's stated goal for voluntary testing, to know how many people lined up against him are infected, is too vague to be of much help. Is the goal of a voluntary testing policy to inform all the participants who exactly on a team is HIV positive? Instead, is the goal to be able to provide players with a statistical figure representing the likelihood of their playing against an HIV-positive athlete? Is the goal to give players who do not want to compete with HIV-positive athletes the opportunity to select other sports in which to participate?

Evidently, an individual making a recommendation needs to indicate clearly what he or she expects to accomplish. Perhaps the most important aspect of making a recommendation is providing reasons or justifications why that recommendation is the right thing to do. Unless the individual making the recommendation explains what he or she hopes to accomplish, others will not be able to evaluate the strength of the justifications, for and against, the proposal. What might be adequate justification for making compiled statistics available to the Centers for Disease Control and Prevention (CDC) may not be at all adequate to justify a policy of publicly identifying individuals who have tested HIV positive.

Being clear about what an individual hopes to accomplish also exhibits that person's central concern. Is that person mostly concerned about himself or herself, for those who have tested HIV positive, for research purposes, or for some other purpose? This may help others spot those cases where a hidden agenda is driving a recommendation. It allows others to assess how well the specifics of the recommendation match up with the stated goals. For instance, the stated goal of a mandatory testing policy may be to identify those people who are HIV positive in order to help them obtain treatment at the earliest possible opportunity. However, if the actual recommendation does not include any counseling component or assistance component, those hearing the recommendation may wonder whether this is truly the genuine goal of the policy.

Furthermore, by clearly stating the goals, individuals can assess the likelihood that the specific recommendation will accomplish the goals and also make comparisons with alternative recommendations for achieving those goals. The other chapters of this textbook explain the types of information (scientific, sociological, legal, historical, and so on) necessary to make such an evaluation.

Justifications for the Recommendations

Ethical deliberation is a process of reasoned argumentation. When a person makes a recommendation about the way things ought to be, that individual is obligated to provide reasons or justifications. Very little in ethics is obvious; very little can be simply assumed. Ethics typically employs two types of justifications: factual and ethical. Mr. Hartman used the first kind of justification when he implied that HIV-positive players could infect other athletes. He compared a football game to a fistfight. He also pointed out that he never played a game in which he did not bleed or have blood on his hands. Mr. Hartman is justifying his recommendation to institute voluntary testing, in part, by saying that infection by players on the field is not merely theoretically possible but, in fact, highly plausible. Of course, even though someone asserts certain claims, he or she may be wrong about the facts of the matter. Others' opinions about a recommendation will therefore depend in part on the strength or weakness of the factual claims put forth to justify it. Again, the rest of the chapters in this text provide some of the information necessary for evaluating the factual claims put forth.

A factual claim by itself, however, is inadequate for accepting an ethical recommendation. After all, this chapter is explaining how to decide what individuals ought to do or think. Therefore, when justifying an ethical recommendation, an individual also employs a particular species of justifications called moral reasons. These differ from economic, legal, scientific, sociological, or psychological reasons. As the author alluded to in the beginning of this chapter, the field of ethics is extremely diverse. No reader should feel surprised that considerable controversy surrounds what constitutes an appropriate moral reason or justification. Many philosophers believe that they can reduce all moral justifications to a single principle. For example, they believe that all moral questions can be settled by ascertaining what will, in the long run, create the greatest amount of overall happiness for all those concerned. Others believe that an ethical inquiry is (or should be) devoted to the development of an individual's own interests. Still others believe that no ethical deliberation can be separated from a religious context. The goal here is to present a framework for conducting ethical deliberations that will be useful to as large an audience as possible. Therefore, the next sections will present four different considerations salient for any substantive ethical deliberation about HIV and sport.

Considerations of Justice.   When a person makes an appeal to justice, he or she is saying that this action is the most fair or that it is the most respectful of others' rights. Fairness simply means that society treats all individuals in similar circumstances alike, without favoritism or prejudice. While the exact nature and extent of rights is controversial, all can probably agree about some of these rights: the right to be free from harm, the right to be free from interference, and the right to develop and pursue one's own life projects. The latter two rights are often grouped together and known as the principle of individual autonomy.

Considerations of Utility.   When appealing to the principle of utility in arguing for a recommendation, a person is claiming that he or she should do whatever action will result in the greatest overall happiness, satisfaction, or benefit of all those involved. This incorporates not just those immediately involved but anyone in the profession or society at large who might have a stake in this decision. Mr. Hartman appeared to be employing some version of this idea in his statement. He asserted that athletes will not play their hardest against competitors who are HIV positive, and this will result in an overall loss to everyone connected with sport; not just the players but the fans as well.

Considerations of Beneficence.   Although some philosophers view beneficence in the rather narrow sense of an obligation to do no harm, most contemporary philosophers interpret it more broadly to include an obligation to help those in need and to promote their welfare where possible. If the voluntary testing policy Mr. Hartman suggested were instituted to help those infected get treatment and counseling, the policy would be justified by appealing to considerations of beneficence.

Considerations of Professional Duties.   Professionals, such as coaches, trainers, physicians, and administrators, take on certain expectations and responsibilities. Frequently, this includes the expectation that professionals have moral duties and responsibilities toward the individuals under their care and have certain special competencies (e.g., knowledge of sports medicine). For example, a team physician may advocate a voluntary testing policy and justify this by an appeal to his or her responsibility for promoting the health of each athlete in her care.

While another philosopher might construct a slightly different list of ethical considerations, these four are a general starting point for most discussions. The descriptions are admittedly sketchy. However, any attempt to expand them takes this chapter further into the field of ethical theory than needed for the stated purposes. When using these principles to justify a recommendation, a person needs to specify exactly how he or she is using the terms. Ethical terms, unlike scientific terms that may be precisely defined, do not necessarily have set meanings that everyone accepts. What some people mean by a right not to be harmed or the extent of a professional obligation may vary somewhat from the way their colleagues use those terms.

Objections to Recommendations

No perfect argument exists. No one can claim absolute certainty that his or her recommendation is right. Therefore, a position will always be provisional, subject to review if the individual encounters new information or new arguments. Those who disagree may present arguments that, like the person's own, are composed of both factual and ethical justifications. However, they may not. They may focus only on challenging the facts in the case. For instance, they may argue that, while considerations of utility are important, an individual's right to privacy should be given greater prominence. Remember that the point of discussing ethical questions with others about HIV and sport is not to win. Rather, it is to reach a conclusion that, all things considered, people believe is the right thing to do. An individual must, therefore, be alert to the weaknesses in his or her own positions. One important way to do this is to listen to opposing positions and carefully consider what opponents are saying. When considering opposing views, apply what philosophers call the principle of charity. The principle of charity requires a person to consider the best possible version of the opponent's view, not the weakest or most easily defeated version. After a person restates and strengthens the opponent's original statement, he or she may then decide to modify or abandon the initial recommendation.

The vexing questions remain about how to balance these considerations, decide which should be given more or less force during deliberations, and determine whether the original recommendation should be endorsed, modified, or rejected. Individuals can use two common sense principles in such deliberations: the principle of consistency and the principle of proportionality. Consistency means that if people reach a conclusion about one case, they should apply the same standard to a similar case. So, if individuals decide, after reflecting on all the facts and weighing ethical considerations, that mandatory testing of college football players ought to be instituted, they would probably be committing to a similar policy for collegiate boxing. Consistency forces individuals to be clear about how much weight they are giving to one ethical consideration and why they have done so. Proportionality means that the more extreme a recommendation is in its scope, the greater the level of justification it requires. If persons recommend a mandatory testing policy for all athletes—high school, college, and professional—regardless of their sport and recommend prohibiting those that test HIV positive, they would need to provide a very strong level of justification. If, however, individuals recommended that basketball players who have blood on their uniforms be pulled from the game until they can put on a clean outfit, they would not need to provide so great a level of justification.

Any discussion about HIV, ethics, and sport should follow these four rules:

1. Specify the details of the recommendation made.
2. Clearly and honestly state the goals of the recommendation.
3. Give ethical and factual justifications for the recommendation.
4. Consider the possible objections to the recommendation.

If the participants in a discussion agree to accept these standards, they will avoid the incoherent, disorganized free-for-all that so often passes for ethical deliberation.

The remainder of this chapter will demonstrate how to use this approach by considering whether HIV-positive boxers ought to be banned from professional boxing. The author chose this issue for three reasons. First, a number of states have been considering passing legislation along these lines, and so the issue is topical. Second, banning professional athletes from their chosen sport is probably the most extreme measure that has been proposed thus far about HIV and sport. Third, the conclusions from this issue can be extrapolated to related questions. If prohibition cannot be justified for boxing, which is by far the most logical candidate, then prohibition will probably not be justifiable for other sports.

Professional Boxing: A Practical Example

Consider the following recommendation: Anyone who tests positive for HIV should be banned from professional boxing. Anyone applying for a license to box in the United States would have to be tested annually, first by an ELISA and then by a repeat of the ELISA and a western blot if the initial test is positive (see chapter 2 for additional information, page 18). The tests would be paid for by the boxer or the boxer's management team as part of the fee. If testing shows the boxer to be HIV positive, he or she would no longer be allowed to box. Moreover, any boxer who fought within the United States with a boxer he or she knows to be HIV positive would forfeit his or her license.

This recommendation seems to meet the first requirement of specificity. It stipulates the kind of athletics (professional boxing), the place (the United States), and provides for a method (mandatory testing) of ascertaining which boxers are, in fact, HIV positive. Furthermore, it specifies what kinds of tests would be used, who would finance them, and how often boxers would be tested. The goal of the recommendation is to prevent athletes who are not HIV positive from becoming infected through contact with HIV-positive boxers.

This recommendation could be justified as follows. Professional boxing is frequently a bloody sport. In many fights, the boxers hit each other hard enough and frequently enough to cause open wounds. Unlike football, which also frequently involves players bleeding, boxers do not have uniforms to prevent topical exposure to blood. Moreover, unlike amateur boxing, professional boxers do not wear headgear, the rounds last longer, professionals fight more rounds, and the referee does not necessarily stop the fight if one of the fighters begins bleeding. Typically, a fight will continue even though a boxer may have an open wound. However, the referee may stop the fight if he or she feels the blood flow is too excessive. This means that both boxers and referees may be repeatedly sprayed with blood throughout a fight. Present research indicates that the HIV virus is transmitted by either blood, semen, or breast milk. Of these, blood seems to be the most critical. The more direct or extensive the blood-to-blood contact, the greater the possibility of successful transmission.

Although no cases have been documented of HIV transmission from an infected boxer to an uninfected one, significantly related cases have occurred. Although they are not common, reports in the medical literature indicate possible infection of medical workers from topical blood exposure (Centers for Disease Control and Prevention 1987), from sports contact between soccer players (Torre, Sampietro, Ferraro, Zeroli, and Speranza 1990), and from fistfights (Ippolito et al. 1994). At present, the number of HIV-positive boxers is not known. The Centers for Disease Control and Prevention, however, reports that a mandatory testing program in Nevada discovered at least two HIV-positive boxers (Springer and Gutskey 1996).

The *Sporting News* reports that a similar program in South Africa found 33 boxers who tested positive (Boxers Test HIV-Positive in South Africa 1995). This means that boxing has an unknown number of HIV-positive athletes. Also, because of the nature of the sport, boxers are at risk of HIV transmission.

The first ethical consideration that supports this recommendation is that a noninfected athlete has a right not to be harmed by another. This may seem like a strange claim for a boxer to make since every boxer voluntarily steps into the ring knowing that the other fighter may be trying to hurt him as much as possible. Estimates vary, but experts conservatively figure that over 400 boxers have died because of boxing-related injuries since 1884 (Futa 1996). However, regarding ethics and sport, two different types of harm are discussed. While athletes are frequently hurt in their sport, they are not harmed in an ethically significant sense. Anyone can be hurt in a football game, baseball game, rugby match, or tennis match for any number of reasons. A clean tackle may break a running back's ankle, or a pitcher may be knocked out by a ball hit directly back at him. In both cases, the athlete has been hurt by the action of another player.

However, consider alternative scenarios in which a batter deliberately lets go of his bat in the direction of the pitcher or a referee ignores dangerous penalties committed by the defense. In such cases, the pitcher or running back is more than simply hurt, he or she has also been harmed. The difference lies, in part, in the intentional violation of mutually agreed upon guidelines, guidelines essential to the original context in which the athletes decided to compete. Athletes weigh the risks of competing in a sport against the pleasure or benefit they will receive from participating. They make their decision whether or not to compete on the basis of this personal assessment. A pitcher may very well have decided not to play baseball if batters, as part of their role, were allowed to intimidate the pitcher by trying to hit him or her with their bat when they are behind the count. A harm, in the morally interesting sense of the word, is when someone damages another and that person neither deserved it nor agreed to permit it.

In other words, a boxer hurt in a fight because of the force of his or her opponent's blow has not been morally harmed. The boxer accepted that being hit is an essential aspect of the sport and was fully aware of the risks involved. However, a fighter who acquires HIV because of the fight has been harmed since this was not a risk he or she agreed to accept in choosing to fight. This means that boxers, promoters, and referees must do what they can to prevent the possible exposure of boxers to HIV within a fight. The surest way to do this is to prevent HIV-positive boxers from fighting.

The second justification for prohibiting HIV-positive boxers from fighting is derived from a combination of utility considerations and the nature of professional boxing. Even if some boxers were willing to fight HIV-positive opponents, the boxing commissions would have to be skeptical about encouraging or allowing such events. If they did, they would be knowingly promoting an event in which a good portion of the audience would be watching out of morbid curiosity to see if the HIV-positive boxer bleeds on the opponent. Allowing such gruesome spectacles hardly seems conducive to creating a more humane and decent society. While some people may find pleasure in watching such events, the overall effect on society would be a coarsening of sensitivities. After all, society does not allow gladiator contests or any other events that will probably lead to the death of one of the participants, even if individuals are willing and eager to participate.

Moreover, allowing such contests would be taking a step backward in the evolution of boxing. Almost all the changes instituted in the 200-year history of boxing (for example, the introduction of gloves, limiting the number of rounds, providing rest breaks, and having referees who can call off a fight if a boxer is in danger) have occurred to decrease the risk of fatality or serious injury. Far from diluting the sport or distorting its essential nature, these alterations have allowed both spectators and participants to focus on what is best in the sport. Advocates of boxing have long argued that what is enjoyable about a good bout is not the prospect of one person killing another but the contest of talents, skills, and heart. Boxing demands endurance, courage, skill, athleticism, intelligence, good strategic and tactical knowledge, patience, and an ability to stay focused under rigorous conditions. These qualities make boxing interesting to watch, not the possibility of one of the contestants dying.

Although plausible reasons exist for barring HIV-positive boxers, the recommendation is unjustified. It has at least four obvious problems. First, it would financially harm HIV-infected boxers by depriving them of their work. Second, it would severely impinge on their privacy and individual autonomy. Third, the arguments for the recommendation rest on dubious claims about further decreasing the risk of transmitting HIV between boxers. Fourth, it would create a false sense of security. Before examining these arguments, recall the principle of proportionality—the greater the stakes, the more stringent the required level of justification. The recommendation goes further than merely demanding mandatory testing for boxers. It calls for a ban on their ability to earn their living without their having done anything to warrant this treatment. Banning boxers for being HIV positive is not the same thing as banning boxers who test positive for drug use. The illicit use of performance-enhancing drugs is an attempt to secure an unfair advantage over an opponent. Fighters who use such drugs abrogate their rights by violating the conditions under which they agreed to fight. Simply being HIV positive constitutes no ethical violation. This means that the recommendation is targeting people who have done nothing wrong. Hence, whatever damage happens to them will count as a harm in the moral sense described earlier.

Since the recommendation specifically targets professional boxers, a positive test would automatically mean the loss of a job and all the problems that this normally entails. Given the cost of medicine and the expense of physicians and hospitals, it is hard to imagine a worse time to lose a job than when facing a life-threatening disease. This loss of income coupled with the very real possibility of losing, or not being eligible for, health insurance means that a boxer might have a hard time securing adequate treatment. This is no small matter since having access to proper treatment may make a significant difference in the quality and quantity of life.

Furthermore, HIV-positive boxers will probably have to endure all this in a very public manner. Theoretically, keeping the results of the test a secret between the individual boxers and the licensing agency might be possible. Perhaps the agency would agree not to reveal the results of the test so long as each HIV-positive boxer immediately agreed to declare the results to be accurate. At a practical level, this seems highly unlikely. No one had any reason to suspect that Arthur Ashe was HIV positive, and yet he was unable to prevent the information from eventually finding its way into the mainstream media. Not only would HIV-positive boxers have to deal with the crushing news that they are HIV-positive, they would have to do so knowing that many other people will know as well. The public exposure that would accompany such news would make an already devastating situation even worse.

However, as arduous as these first two problems might be, being forced to quit may be even more devastating to a boxer's sense of self. People seldom become professional boxers on a whim; it takes years of training, dedication, and sacrifice. As a result of this enormous personal investment, much of a boxer's identity may be wrapped up in his or her career. Countless numbers of champions have appeared satisfied with their triumphs and retired with their health intact. The drive that made them compete all those years, however, keeps them coming back for just one more fight. Society places a high premium on protecting individual autonomy. An essential aspect of this right is all people being free to choose their life's work, to pursue their dreams, to develop their skills and talents to their fullest potential, and to shape their destinies. No one has the right to succeed, but all have the right to be free to try.

Still, do these considerations outweigh the right of the uninfected boxers not to be harmed? As dreadful as the publicity, loss of job, and subsequent difficulties might be for the infected boxers, they must be set beside the possibly fatal consequences for the uninfected boxers. To settle this, the readers need to be clear about what exactly the risk is of infection by one boxer to another in a bout. The American Academy of Pediatrics Committee on Sports Medicine and Fitness (1991), the World Health Organization Consensus Statement—Consultation on AIDS and Sports (1992), the Canadian Academy of Sports Medicine Task Force on Infectious Disease in Sports (1993), and the National Collegiate Athletic Association (NCAA) (1992) have all concluded that the risk of infection by one athlete to another (even in contact sports such as football, boxing, and wrestling) is not sufficient to warrant a policy of mandatory testing. Dr. Anthony Fauci, one of the country's leading AIDS researchers and director of the National Institute of Allergy and Infectious Diseases, and Dr. Michael Johnson, head of the AIDS education program for the NBA Players Association, have both argued that the risk of one athlete passing the infection on in the course of an athletic event is so unlikely that it is nearly impossible to measure (*Nightline* 1996). One study (Brown et al. 1995) calculated that the convergence of factors required to transmit HIV successfully from one athlete to another in a football game is less than 1 per 85 million game contacts.

These recommendations are supported by the medical literature about hepatitis B virus (HBV), which is far more resilient and stable than HIV. No case of a sport-related HBV infection in the United States has been reported to the CDC. However, one episode occurred in 1980 in Japan; a sumo wrestler infected his opponent (Mast et al. 1995). Some might argue that the number of people with HIV is much higher than those infected with HBV, and hence the danger is substantially greater. While definitive data about the actual number of HIV-positive boxers in the United States does not exist, the figure is probably quite small. Despite all the attention focused on boxer Tommy Morrison's condition, only one other boxer has tested positive (out of 2,100 tested) in Nevada since 1988 when the state began its policy (Springer and Gutskey 1996). In a yearlong survey of NCAA member institutions, only 12 of the 548 responding schools reported having any HIV-positive or AIDS-diagnosed athletes (McGrew et al. 1993). These figures are not enough to establish the rate of infection among professional boxers conclusively. Additionally, readers need to recognize that the chapter is not discussing a high-risk population, such as intravenous drug users.

Some may still argue that, even though these risks are admittedly small, since something can be done to protect uninfected boxers, it ought to be done. However, alternatives to the recommendation would reduce the already negligible risk even further and not penalize infected boxers. Since one of the conditions for transmitting HIV from one boxer to another is for both parties to have open cuts, ways of reducing bleeding during boxing matches should be studied. The most obvious solution is to have professional boxing adopt many of the same guidelines that now govern amateur boxing, particularly the introduction of headgear. Having all fighters wear headgear would significantly reduce the amount of cuts and abrasions that take place in a fight since it protects the area most likely to be cut, the face. Moreover, having professional boxers wear headgear has been advocated by many physicians for years for health reasons entirely unrelated to HIV. The vast majority of damage done to boxers, both in terms of fatalities and long-term health problems, results from head injuries. As Dr. David Hovda, head of the University of California at Los Angeles' neuroscience department and a specialist in severe brain injuries, puts it,

> I know it's not artistic; it may or may not hurt the sport's popularity to some degree, but I can't emphasize enough the importance of headgear. The whole principle of having headgear is to add to the types of protection that we don't have to begin with. If I could do it, I would have everyone wear headgear. (Futa 1996)

Although the introduction of headgear would be challenged by many boxing enthusiasts as an intolerable dilution of boxing, the sport has been altered a number of times over the years to increase the safety of boxers.

Finally, utility considerations also argue against the recommendation. It may reassure a large majority of boxers that they are now safe because they will not face HIV-positive fighters, but this reassurance would be deceptive and possibly counterproductive. The way that athletes are most likely to become infected is the same way as anyone else: through unprotected sex or the sharing of needles. Banning HIV-positive boxers would shift the focus away from these activities where the risk of infection is genuine and where athletes actually have some measure of control over the dangers. A ban could delude boxers into thinking that they are protected from HIV. Moreover, instituting such a policy would say to the public at large that the likelihood of passing HIV from one fighter to another is strong enough to warrant stripping fighters of their licenses to box, even though the scientific data does not support such a claim. This would mislead the public about the nature of HIV and further contribute to the climate of fear, irrationality, and prejudice that as professionals and policy makers, the readers should be trying to combat.

For all these reasons, the author would argue against the original recommendation of banning HIV-positive athletes from professional boxing. All of the points raised against banning HIV-positive boxers rest, in large part, on the empirical data about the possibility of transmission from one boxer to another. If evidence showed that amateur boxers were infecting each other with HIV (or similar viruses), the context of these objections would alter.

Conclusion and Recommendations

This chapter has presented a framework for exploring ethical questions regarding HIV and sport and has shown how to use this framework in practice. Even so, many readers may reason that the chapter has left out critical distinctions or facts that ought to be stated before deciding about a ban on HIV-positive individuals in boxing; this is as it should be. Ethical deliberation is an ongoing process. All conclusions are open to review and debate. Consequently, as mentioned previously, this process may strike some people as a frustrating quagmire.

Frustrating as it may be, however, the process of ethical inquiry does bring its rewards. Framing and developing the discussion, as in the manner used here, helps clarify and refine individuals' thinking. This, in turn, contributes to a deeper understanding of the issues and persons' own ethical commitments. Respectful, though rigorous, argumentation also shows respect for those who disagree. Few are moral monsters. Coherent ethical inquiry can emphasize shared commitments as well as points of dispute. This is important because it preserves the integrity of the moral community. It demonstrates that society is, by and large, committed to developing what ought to be. Viewed from this perspective, conducting thoughtful and thorough ethical investigations into topics such as HIV and sport are essential, even though they may seldom be easy.

References

33 Boxers Test HIV-Positive in South Africa. (1995, July 17). *Sporting News,* p. 33. Retrieved October 15, 1998 from the World Wide Web: **http://www3.nando.net/ newsroom/sports/oth/1995/oth/box/feat/archive/071795/box29022.html**

American Academy of Pediatrics Committee on Sports Medicine and Fitness. (1991). Human immunodeficiency virus [acquired immunodeficiency syndrome (AIDS) virus] in the athletic setting. *Pediatrics, 88* (3), 640–41.

Brown, L., Jr., Phillips, D., Chu, A., Brown, C., Jr., & Knowlan, D., Jr. (1995). Bleeding injuries in professional football: Estimating the risk for HIV transmission. *Annals of Internal Medicine, 122* (4), 271–74.

Calabrese, L. H., Haupt, H.A., Hartman, L., Strauss, R.H. (1993). HIV and sports: What is the risk? *Sports Medicine Update, 21*(3), 173–80.

Canadian Academy of Sports Medicine Task Force on Infectious Disease in Sports. (1993). HIV as it relates to sports. *Clinical Journal of Sports Medicine, 3,* 63–65.

Centers for Disease Control and Prevention. (1987). Update: Human immunodeficiency virus infections in health care workers exposed to the blood of infected patients. *Morbidity and Mortality Weekly Reports, 36* (19), 285–89.

Futa, D. (1996). Boxing: An interview with an expert. *Rawley Valverde AT THE HACIENDA.* Channel One .com Online Network. Retrieved August 1, 1997 from the World Wide Web: **http://www.channelone.com/ns/news/96/04/960429/ story1.html**

Ippolito, G., Del Poggio, P., Arici, C., Gregis, G.P., Antomilli, G., Riva, E., & Dianzani, F. (1994). Transmission of zidovudine-resistant HIV during a bloody fight. *Journal of the American Medical Association, 272* (6), 433–34.

Mast, E.E., Goodman, R.A., Bond, W.W., Bavero, M.S., & Drotman, P.D. (1995). Transmission of bloodborne pathogens during sports: Risk and prevention. *Annals of Internal Medicine, 122* (4), 283–85.

McGrew, C., Dick, R.W., Schniedwind, K., & Gikas, P. (1993). Survey of NCAA institutions concerning HIV/AIDS policies and universal precautions. *Medicine and Science in Sports and Exercise, 25* (8), 917–21.

National Collegiate Athletic Association. (1992–1993). *NCAA Sports Medicine Handbook. AIDS and intercollegiate athletics (pp.24–25). Guideline 2-H.* Overland Park, KS: National Collegiate Athletic Association.

Nightline. (1996). Television program, produced by Tom Bettag. February 13. ABC. Washington, D.C.

Springer, S. & Gutskey, E. (1996, February 13). Boxer's HIV wouldn't have been detected in California. *Los Angeles Times—Washington Edition,* p. A1. Retrieved August 1, 1997 from the World Wide Web: **http://www.ama-assn.org/special/hiv/newsline/current/today/cdctemp.htm#box**

Torre, D., Sampietro, C., Ferraro, G., Zeroli, C., & Speranza, F. (1990). Transmission of HIV-1 infection via sports injury (Letter). *Lancet, 335* (8697), 1105.

World Health Organization Consensus Statement—Consultation on AIDS and Sports. (1992). *Journal of the American Medical Association, 267* (10), 1312–14.

CHAPTER 8

HIV, Ethics, and the Sport Practitioner

Jennifer M. Beller
Eastern Michigan University, and Affiliate Faculty, The Center for ETHICS,
University of Idaho

Sharon Kay Stoll
Director, The Center for ETHICS, University of Idaho

Bud is the athletic trainer at Big Time University. He works closely day-to-day with many athletes on the men's basketball team. They consider Bud one of the boys and do not appear inhibited with how they talk around Bud. In fact, Bud hears conversations about wild parties with alcohol, sex, and so forth. Some of the athletes talk about keeping score, seeing how many women they can sleep with in a row without sleeping with the same one twice. Bud is concerned about these young men, their apparent lack of concern about their personal conduct, and the potential for spreading sexually transmitted diseases (STDs). Yet, Bud realizes the athletic department has a series of seminars about alcohol, date rape, sex, and social responsibility. He figures that these should help people become more responsible.

The team doctor, Doc Fix-It, tells Bud that he has seen and tested much of the team for some form of STDs. In fact, he says that 15% have tested positive on more than one occasion. In a private conversation, he tells Bud that Mike, the leading scorer, tested positive for human immunodeficiency virus (HIV). Doc Fix-It also tells Bud that Mike is under medical supervision, seeing a counselor for help with the emotional devastation of the disease, and appears to have no medical problems that preclude his participation at this time. Doc Fix-It informs Bud that he is telling him this information as a favor so that when Bud has to work with Mike, Bud can take extra precautions. Bud is in a quandary. He knows that other trainers must also work with Mike. However, Doc Fix-It told him the information in confidence, and so Bud is not sure if he should tell the others. Bud begins to weigh the pros and cons. He reads his professional code of ethics and finds no specific information concerning confidentiality and disclosure. Thus, he decides to have a confidential meeting with the student trainers about safety precautions to take while working with Mike based on the National Collegiate Athletic Association (NCAA) *Guideline 2-H* (1994).

Somehow, rumors surface around the training room and the athletic arena that Mike is HIV positive. Doc Fix-It confronts Bud and accuses him of violating a confidence and therefore unjustifiably hurting Mike. Bud knows the damage has already occurred. However, he feels unsure about how to proceed because many people outwardly claim that they do not have a problem working with Mike or playing on the same team. At the same time, some athletic trainers avoid working with Mike, and athletes keep their distance. Bud decides that he needs to seek legal advice from the university counsel to see if he did the right thing. He calls the university counsel, Mr. Right, and is told that the university does not have a specific policy concerning disclosure of an HIV-infected individual. Mr. Right does state that according to the courts, the issue of disclosure is based on whether by not disclosing the information, individuals will be placed at significant risk. Furthermore, Mr. Right refers Bud to the state law that states that very few incidences exist in which disclosure becomes necessary.

The word spreads, however, and the media picks up Mike's story. Mike decides to address the rumors and announces that he is HIV positive. He also says that he is taking all the precautions necessary and keeping himself physically fit. The team doctor also attests to the fact that Mike is capable of playing at this point in his career without experiencing adverse side effects. However, players and coaches on some teams do not want to play the team unless Mike is not allowed to play.

Bud knows that their concerns are based on misinformation about how the disease spreads and on hysteria borne out of ignorance. No amount of discussion seems to

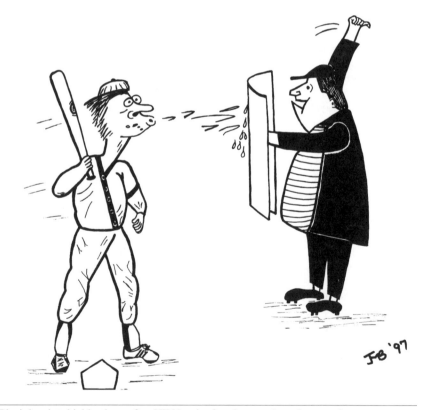

Plexiglas riot shields: the perfect HIV barrier for players who spit at umpires.
Illustration by Jennifer Beller.

dissuade these coaches and players in their goal to remove Mike from eligibility. Bud wonders whether he did the right thing—did Bud correctly address each alternative choice as it arose? Did Bud do the right thing when he learned about Mike's condition? Should he have done anything differently when Doc Fix-It confided in him? Should Bud have behaved differently when dealing with Mike? Should Bud have educated his athletes about blood-borne pathogens earlier and better than he did?

Ethics and HIV/AIDS

How, as in this athletic trainer's case, can one identify moral issues and decide if actions are or are not morally appropriate? Athletic trainers and sport practitioners, in the normal routine of their jobs, face this scenario and many other similar situations. Some may argue that because the potential ramifications of disease transmission are so great, all have a right to know that a player is HIV positive. On the other hand, others may argue that the athletic trainer acted immorally by breaching trust and confidentiality. Still others may argue that this is not a moral problem but rather a legal issue that should be settled by the courts. Some readers may have referenced their professional code of ethics to see what this athletic trainer should have done. Perhaps other readers have no idea what to do and figure that until it happens to them, it is none of their concern.

How people address moral issues in their lives reflects their understanding of ethics, morality, values, and principles in relation to others. To begin, individuals must learn to examine the issues and questions involved through an impartial, reflective, and consistent reasoning process (Fox and DeMarco 1990). In other words, people must step back from the issue, attempt to examine all facets of the issue, and avoid letting their emotions dictate their decisions. The process requires both getting the facts straight and keeping their minds clear (Frankena 1973). Second, individuals cannot answer these questions by simply appealing to what people generally think. Social belief and action have been known to be morally wrong. Individuals must attempt to find answers based on sound reasoning, good judgment, and universal principles tempered by historical fact and cultural tradition that they themselves regard as correct. This process requires that people think for themselves and not follow herd behavior, as described by Karl Marx. When individuals make moral decisions, those decisions must come from a principled, reasoned perspective. This perspective should be honed, tempered, and based on the knowledge of what is historically and ethically known to be right and good.

The Australian Olympic team's response to playing a U.S. team containing Earvin "Magic" Johnson indicates that ignorance and oftentimes hysteria exist in relation to HIV and its potential risk of transmission. Yet, the ethical issues surrounding HIV/AIDS are varied and diverse. Moral questions about HIV/AIDS in sport concern testing, disclosure, informed consent, confidentiality, rights, obligations, and risks, to name a few. The study of ethics is often considered nebulous and esoteric. However, the purpose of this chapter is to provide a practical framework from which the reader can examine his or her personal values and beliefs in relation to the professional issues faced by a sports medicine professional. More specifically, the following questions will be examined:

- What is ethics?
- What is the relationship between ethics and the law?
- What is personal morality?
- How does personal morality relate to professional practice for sport practitioners, especially in relation to the issues surrounding HIV/AIDS?

What the authors advocate in this chapter is beyond the scope of moral training. Moral training implies the drilling of rules and acceptable behaviors without encouraging understanding of the principles involved. The authors' goal is not only to help develop and encourage the capacity to make moral judgments but to inspire readers to have courage to act upon what they learn (Kohlberg 1981). More specifically, the authors' goal is that the readers learn to reflect on current moral issues in light of fundamental moral principles, make rational judgments, and translate those beliefs into appropriate moral action. The next section will explain some basic terminology and concepts.

What Are Ethics and Morality?

Classical ethics, in its purest sense, is the theoretical study of right and wrong, good and evil. It studies the how and the who of different historical theories (Stoll and Beller 1994). Ethicists study great writers from Plato to Kant, Bentham to Mill, Augustine to Neibur. The purpose of the classical study of ethics is to provide a background, backdrop, and perspective of what the great thinkers believed was the right and the wrong of human behavior. The great writers challenge people to think, argue, debate, and wonder. Classical ethics is important and even imperative to understand the nature of morality. However, the first and continuing goal, whether studying the classics or practicing applied ethics, should be a personal quest to understand one's own values and beliefs.

Morality is concerned with one's actions, intentions, and motives as they affect and impinge on others (Lumpkin, Stoll, and Beller 1995). Morality concerns personal beliefs and actions and exhibiting how individuals value interpersonal relationships. A value is something of relative worth. The key is the word *relative*. In other words, what one person might value another might see as having little value. What one person values in a nonmoral sense is different than what another values.

Two general categories of values come into play: nonmoral and moral. Nonmoral values are usually extrinsically based or things such as winning, fame, prestige, money, power, and position. "They are not moral in the sense that they are not people, intentions, motives, deeds, or traits of character that affect other persons" (Lumpkin, Stoll and Beller, 1995). Nonmoral goods guide how individuals make moral decisions. For example, if an individual values winning more than honesty, he or she can more easily violate the value of honesty and the trust of another. In other words, the value to win drives the moral action.

Moral values are the relative worth one places on some type of virtuous behavior. They are internal, subjective and immeasurable in an objective sense (Lumpkin, Stoll, and Beller 1995). They are traits or dispositions that individuals esteem or portray. Without moral values, having interpersonal relationships would be difficult. Examples of moral values include respect, honesty, responsibility, justice, and beneficence. One of the goals of ethical and moral reasoning should be to think about the few moral values that are important, rank those values, and then decide if any mitigating circumstances would violate the stated moral value. Understand, however, that a value should be violated by only a few exceptions, that the violation can occur only in relation to another moral value, and that people should not base their decisions on personal interest.

When deciding about moral values, principles called first rules are written. These first rules are universal guides that tell individuals "which kinds of actions, intentions, and motives are prohibited, obligatory, or permitted in human interactions" (Lumpkin, Stoll, and Beller 1995). Generally, because one knows more easily when a moral value is violated, principles are written in the negative. In other words, if a person values honesty, the principle or first rule is, "I will not lie, cheat, or steal." By placing moral values into a universal form, such as principles, standards exist against which to measure tough decisions.

Developing a comprehensive set of principles is no easy task. It requires much thought, musing, and questioning of self, past history, present social conditions, and universal concepts of right and wrong. Once implementing this process, one must apply and challenge those beliefs and values in everyday life. Only then can a person examine what the great writers have said and have it make meaning in his or her personal and professional worlds.

Although the terms ethics and morality are often used interchangeably, they are not the same. Morality, as opposed to ethics, is one's actions, intentions, and motives as they affect and impinge upon others (Lumpkin, Stoll, and Beller 1995). In its most general form, morality is common decency toward others. It involves having consideration and concern for others as well as ourselves. Morality also attempts to determine right from wrong and good from bad. Morality, as practiced in its theoretical sense, is actual personal behavior, associated with moral values and principles, directed toward others. These moral values and principles need to be evaluated, understood, and fleshed out before an individual chooses or engages in a particular course of action.

As noted earlier, the moral values cited most often are concerned with making ethical decisions about honesty, fairness, and respect. (DeGeorge 1990; Frankena 1973; Lumpkin, Stoll, and Beller 1995; Stoll and Beller 1994). These values are the cornerstone of most of the world's great religions, the Judeo-Christian tradition, the Jeffersonian democracy, and the U.S. Constitution. Without these values and the accompanying principles, society would be in chaos. We, as a people, would not be able to buy and sell, make contracts, do business, own property, have peace, live in freedom, or pursue happiness. Principles, per se, are the actual written statements exemplifying the moral values of an individual, group, or society.

In the present scenario with Bud and Mike, the dilemma begins and ends with Bud's inability to make an informed and personal moral decision about the case in hand. If Bud had fleshed out his personal values and developed a set of principles, perhaps all the ethical questions may not have arisen. If Bud had a good sense about his principles, maybe he would have forced the university to write a better policy statement about blood-borne pathogens. If he had understood the importance of honesty, fairness, and respect, he would have caused a comprehensive educational program to be in place before this incident occurred. Bud knew the existing education program was not effective, and he knew that athletes were practicing unsafe sex. He also knew that the athletes apparently believed they were immortal. They had a "that won't happen to me" mentality. Research literature, the press, and the behavior of these athletes gave Bud enough evidence to prove to even the most stubborn athlete that a problem exists and is not going away. Many knew that these athletes practice risky behavior–both Doc Fix-It and Bud knew. However, Doc Fix-It decided to pass responsibility to the athletic department. Bud had his head in the sand and ignored the possible problems until a situation arose.

Bud, as all trainers and educators, has a responsibility to tell his clients and students the truth about infectious diseases early and often. He has a responsibility to educate them about proper protective behavior to avoid contracting HIV/AIDS as well as moral conduct to practice when another is infected. Passive education, in this scenario, was not working. The athletes in question needed intervention education. This directly challenges athletes about their values and sexual practices. Athletes need to be engaged in direct and confrontational discussions about HIV/AIDS and their own practices. This sort of education is not a one-time-only procedure. Intervention education must occur often and continuously to support higher-order reasoning about life's current dilemmas. Short, one-time "lectures" that tell athletes what to do and not to do are ineffective. Nancy Reagan's "Just Say No" campaign underscored the shortsightedness of such a strategy. Foresight and active intervention education are the keys to solving this moral dilemma. Unfortunately, in this scenario, comprehensive education, both medical and moral, was lacking from the beginning and foresight was lost or never existed.

How Can Individuals Use Professional Ethical Codes?

Professional ethics are the stated professional principles—codes—that each organization deems important. They generally are rules of moral action within the organization. An organization develops these codes based on some perceived moral conduct deemed imperative to the professional process (Stoll and Beller 1994). Although most sport-related disciplines and organizations (for example, the National Athletic Trainers Association [NATA], the National Association for Sport and Physical Education [NASPE], the American Medical Association [AMA], and the American College of Sports Medicine [ACSM]) have specific codes for their members, most professional codes have similar purposes (DeGeorge 1990).

- Codes detail guidelines about client and professional behavior.
- Codes set standards for interpersonal, client, and professional behavior.
- Codes monitor professional behavior.
- Codes detail how to report and adjudicate questionable behavior.

Professional codes are not self-serving but rather regulative. They protect public interests and those they serve. Professional codes are specific and honest. They set standards by which to monitor organization members. By following codes, individuals are expected to set an example of proper conduct, refrain from improper conduct, and be known for refraining from such improper conduct. Because codes are not law but rather general guidelines, violations generally involve censure or expulsion of members.

Professional codes have useful purposes. They force large numbers of individuals to think through their mission and the importance and obligations that they as a group and as individuals have to the discipline, to each other, and to their respective clients. Once adopted, codes can be used to generate continuing discussions of the codes and inculcate new members in their field to develop professional virtues. These codes can act as a ready guide to help make decisions and assure the organization, public, and others that the profession has a touchstone by which to measure ethical actions.

These codes, though, are only a small piece in the total educational picture. Codes do not guarantee an individual's moral action, that a profession or discipline serves the public, or prevent the organization's members from acting unethically. In general, codes are only as useful as the education available about those codes and the active role of members in policing themselves. The goal of this chapter, though, is not specifically to address professional ethics. That is the role of the reader's particular professional society. Rather, this chapter addresses individual moral behavior as it relates to personal and professional ethics.

Bud researched his professional code of ethics and remained confidential in the scenario, though he probably was naive about what confidentiality means to his young athletic trainers. Attorneys, physicians, and psychiatrists are professionals bound by codes of confidentiality, which their respective professions' professional code of ethics specifically details. In some cases, if a professional violates confidentiality as described in his or her profession's codes, censure or legal ramifications may result. Sport practitioners and athletic trainers are not bound to codes of confidentiality. That does not mean, however, that confidentiality is not important to this work and the relationships formed with clients.

Confidentiality implies that discussions and communications, both written and verbal, are not publicly disseminated (Beller and Stoll 1995). If an individual is considered a confidant, he or she can be trusted. That person can know conversations, discussions, and privileged information and will not share this with others. Hand in hand with confidentiality is the moral value of honesty. Honesty implies that an individual is trustworthy, open, and reliable toward another. Yet, this openness does not imply that an individual should share all conversations and communications with others. If a confidant believes in the value of honesty and the tenets of confidentiality, that person must know what information is confidential, when to hold information in confidence, and when to share information. If a person has established values and principles ahead of time, although situations at times may be difficult, that person has a framework from which to make consistent, impartial, and reflective decisions to guide moral actions.

With the example given in this chapter, what values and principles of confidentiality may have been violated? Could Bud, as an athletic trainer, have handled this situation in a better way? In this case, Doc Fix-It assumed confidentiality when discussing Mike with Bud. Oftentimes in society, a conversation is assumed to be confidential because of someone's position and/or because the discussion occurred in private. Perhaps, Doc Fix-It unknowingly assumed that Bud, as a trainer, held to the same codes of confidentiality that he enjoys through the AMA. However, one should never assume confidentiality. In cases where communications should be held in confidence, the individual providing the confidential information should ask ahead of time, "Is this conversation in confidence? What does confidence mean to you?" Based on the answers, the person can then decide whether to share the information and if the listener will hold it in mutual confidence. In Bud's case, as the trainer, this quandary may have several solutions that do not violate confidentiality about Mike.

The issue of how others treat Mike because of his HIV status involves respect. This entails treating others how we ourselves would want to be treated. In other words, do individuals act consistently? Can their actions be applied to similar circumstances (Stoll and Beller 1995)? Not only do individuals have a personal obligation to treat others with respect but professional obligations exist, as well. Thus, how people treat one individual should be how they treat all individuals. Historically, purely by being part of a certain group, class, and/or race, individuals have been treated poorly. Often, individuals can rationalize behaviors because they are part of the social norm. Kretchmar (1994) calls this behavior moral callousness, whereby people are insensitive to others and rationalize their actions because others do it.

In Mike's case, possibly because of hysteria and ignorance, he is being treated poorly. Head trainers are responsible for developing a collegial environment that deals with issues in an honest, confidential, and forthright manner. All individuals should be treated with dignity and respect. The reader's task may not be easy. Dealing with ignorance, hysteria, and moral callousness is a long-term process involving educational programs concerning HIV/AIDS and interactive dialogues about common decency and respect. This process culminates with continually demonstrating, with actions, that all individuals should be treated with respect.

However, if individuals want confidentiality, educators must teach the meaning and value of it. In today's society, the practice of honor and integrity is hard to find. In fact, few understand the meaning of these terms. Honor is the practice of holding to one's principles, while integrity means being above corruption. If one has honor, that person follows a very specific set of personal and/or professional principles. One has integrity when others know that the person has not defiled his or her honor. A few institutions in America still practice and support the concepts of honor and integrity. At the United States Military Academy at West Point, the United States Naval Academy at Annapolis, and the United States Air Force Academy at Colorado Springs, the faculty and students understand the importance of learning these two precepts. At all three institutions, formal and informal education is specifically directed toward character education. Unfortunately, even there, the education system sometimes fails. If we as a society want young people today to practice confidentiality, be honorable, and have unquestionable integrity, educational programs must teach them about the meaning of honor, integrity, and confidentiality. If sports medicine wishes confidentiality to be successful, the ethics educational module must be the most important facet of the general curriculum. To paraphrase a piece written by one of the founders of the ethical movement in sport, Earle Zeigler

(1984), the sole most important practice and education in sport today is ethics.

To put this into practice, athletic trainers and sports professionals must first realize that medical diagnoses and problems are confidential—between that person and the athlete. Bud acted naively by speaking with the student trainers. He had a responsibility to be concerned for their safety when dealing with blood-borne pathogens. However, to believe that they would keep the information confidential showed a complete lack of understanding of human behavior. Bud was responsible for the rumors about Mike. Bud may have done the right thing in warning the student trainers. However, his action is questionable considering his supposedly confidential discussion with Doc Fix-It and his responsibility to Mike.

Instead, Bud should have retrained all student trainers about blood-borne diseases, using the NCAA *Guideline 2-H* (1994) and Occupational Safety and Health Administration (OSHA) guidelines (1992). He should have demanded that they treat every athlete with the same competent procedures. As a head trainer, Bud could have held seminars with the student trainers and spent time discussing proper techniques, practices, and safety precautions when working with any athlete and reviewing how diseases are transmitted.

Bud has the responsibility of making these standard operating procedures practiced every moment of the training day. Every athlete should be considered a risk. Every trainer is obligated to self and society to take precautions.

Bud showed his own lack of reasoning and obligation to the client/professional confidentiality code when he singled out Mike. Just because Mike is HIV positive does not mean that he loses his rights as an individual. Bud's behavior also underscores the importance of active intervention, moral education, and character education. Bud may be the professional in this case, but he acted highly unprofessionally. Bud, as all professionals, should also be involved in ethics education.

What Is the Relationship Between Ethics and the Law?

Probably due to the current litigious society, much of the literature concerning AIDS/HIV discusses what is morally right in legal terms (Burris, Dalton, and Miller 1993; Dalton and Burris 1987; McKenzie 1991; O'Malley 1989). In a legal sense, the standard of correct conduct toward another individual or group of individuals is based on socialized ethics. These laws, developed by the people, are based on society's perceptions of what is right and wrong. In the case of HIV/AIDS, perceptions involve sensory experiences to achieve an understanding about some issue, standard, or act of correct conduct. An individual has perceptions. However, in the case of laws, perception involves a collective conscious. Perception, though, with its standard framed from only a personal view, can be very biased. As such, it can involve little or no reasoning or critical thinking.

In contrast, ethics is the overarching umbrella of correct conduct. In other words, ethics is a higher and broader standard than the legal precedent of socialized ethics—the law. With ethics, rightness and wrongness are based on personal values, principles, and their relationship to others.

Making and using guidelines, such as laws, as the basis of right conduct and human decency can be very shortsighted, naive, and problematic. Many specific examples throughout history demonstrate that the social conscious, in this case laws, can be morally wrong. For instance, the United States had laws (Jim Crow laws and slavery) that morally violated individuals' rights and human decency. Adolph Hitler's ability to change the social conscious is another classic example where laws were morally wrong. In these cases, individuals, purely by being a part of a certain class of people, were treated with less worth than others. Thus, while laws provide a general framework, they have limitations when using them as standards from which to decide all right conduct. In other words, people must look beyond the laws to a set of values and universal principles.

Bud went to the laws and even to the university counsel, Mr. Right, to find resolution to his dilemma. Unfortunately, he found no moral support. The law gave parameters about the meaning of justice. The law underscored the importance of treating Mike fairly as well as protecting the rights of others. Bud was reasonable in contacting the attorney. However, his action was a day late and a dollar short. Again, Bud should have realized earlier that a policy needs to be supported by the laws of society. He should have known the legal parameters of this situation before it occurred. Unfortunately, Bud's actions are common in our litigious society. After a problem occurs, people contact attorneys to find out if they did the right thing. The laws are developed to support the social ethics of a society, and they should be considered. However, laws will not guide reasonable development of professional conduct. Bud and the rest of Big Time University's faculty and staff should have already had a comprehensive policy and guidelines in place to deal with this impending problem. They should have known that the university and one of its employees would face this situation sooner or later.

Conclusion and Recommendations

Addressing the weighty moral issues in life is a difficult task. Many factors, influences, and value systems come into play. Professionals have the task of sorting out the fact from fiction, understanding their personal values and beliefs, developing daily principles to guide their lives, and having the courage to take a stand. As Dietrich Bonhoeffer stated, "It is not the evil people in the world that are a problem, it is the good people who do not have the courage to take a stand on what is right" (Sereny 1995).

Bud's ethical dilemma lies in two first principles: I will not lie, cheat, or steal; and I will not be disrespectful of others. A major professional code of conduct or rule also surfaced—the issue of confidentiality. As this chapter has discussed, Bud violated professional principles. He was not honest, and he was definitely disrespectful. Doc Fix-It did not help, nor did the university counsel. Bud was stuck with his own lack of moral knowledge and fumbled along until Mike was thoroughly violated.

When deciding what to do when ethics and morality surface, the best course of action is education. Preliminary intervention, ethical educational programs directed toward the study of ethics and morals in life and society, are sorely needed. Many of Bud's problems occurred because of lack of foresight in program development and applied ethics. Bud would have fared better if he and other trainers had received active moral education. This should have included intervention programs in place for self, student trainers, and athletes.

The social issue of being HIV positive deals with a health-related problem that will not go away soon. However, with medical and moral education, sports medicine professions can make reasoned decisions in which no one—the athlete, the competitor, or the practicing trainer—will be placed into medical or ethical jeopardy.

References

Beller, J.M., & Stoll, S.K. (1995). Professional honesty and confidentiality. *Strategies, 9* (3), 13–15.

Burris, S., Dalton, H.L., & Miller, J.L. (1993). *AIDS and the Law Today: A New Guide for The Public.* New Haven, CT: Yale University Press.

Dalton, H.L., & Burris, S. (1987). *AIDS and the Law.* New Haven, CT: Yale University Press.

DeGeorge, R.T. (1990). *Business Ethics* (3rd ed.). New York: Macmillan.

Fox, R.M., & DeMarco, J.P. (1990). *Moral Reasoning: A Philosophic Approach to Applied Ethics.* Fort Worth, TX: Holt, Rinehart & Winston.

Frankena, W. (1973). *Ethics* (2nd ed.). Englewood Cliffs, NJ: Prentice Hall.

Kohlberg, L. (1981). *The Philosophy of Moral Development: Moral Stages and the Idea of Justice.* New York: Harper & Row.

Kretchmar, R.S. (1994). *Practical Philosophy of Sport.* Champaign, IL: Human Kinetics.

Lumpkin, A., Stoll, S.K., & Beller, J.M. (1995). *Sport Ethics: Applications for Fair Play.* St. Louis: Mosby.

McKenzie, N.F. (1991). *The AIDS Reader: Social, Political, Ethical Issues.* New York: Meridian Books.

National Collegiate Athletic Association. (1993–1994). *Guideline 2-H. Bloodborne Pathogens and Intercollegiate Athletics. NCAA Sports Medicine Handbook.* Overland Park, KS: National Collegiate Athletic Association, 24–28.

Occupational Safety and Health Administration. (1992). *Bloodborne Pathogens* (Standards—29 CFR). Washington, DC: U.S. Document Service, Directorate of Safety and Directorate of Health.

O'Malley, P. (1989). *The AIDS Epidemic: Private Rights and the Public Interest.* Boston: Beacon Press.

Sereny, G. (1995). *Albert Spear's Battle with the Truth.* New York: Knopf.

Stoll, S.K., & Beller, J.M. (1994). *Moral Education: What It Is and Is Not.* Unpublished manuscript, The Center for ETHICS*, University of Idaho, Moscow, ID.

Stoll, S.K., & Beller, J.M. (1995). Professional respect—make it universal. *Strategies, 8* (7). 27–29.

Zeigler, E. (1984). *Ethics and Morality in Sport and Physical Education: an Experimental Approach.* Champaign, IL: Stipes Publishing Company.

CHAPTER 9

Legal Issues Pertaining to HIV in Sport

Mary A. Hums
University of Louisville, Kentucky

Two boxers go toe-to-toe in a heavyweight matchup. A quarterback takes a forearm to the chin and gets sacked. A shortstop gets spiked turning a double play. Cyclists form a pileup after crashing during a sprint race. A pool deck cuts a swimmer's foot. In each instance, blood is present, and a coach, trainer, or perhaps another athlete may become involved. The involvement of HIV-positive individuals in sport presents sport management policy makers with numerous dilemmas. When making decisions and formulating organizational policy, sport managers must examine the social, legal, ethical, economic, political, and educational considerations related to their decisions.

Legislation

This chapter specifically deals with the legal issues sport managers and trainers must face when framing organizational policies involving HIV-positive individuals' opportunities to participate in sport or be employed in the sport industry. It will first discuss information about legislation relevant to people with disabilities in general. Then it will describe how that legislation applies to HIV-positive persons.

Disability Status

An HIV-positive person is, by law, considered a person with a disability. As such, someone who is HIV positive is provided with all the protections under the appropriate laws that any person with a disability would have. The major pieces of legislation dealing with people with disabilities that sport managers and trainers need to be educated about are Section 504 of the Rehabilitation Act of 1973 and the Americans With Disabilities Act (ADA) of 1990.

Section 504 of the Rehabilitation Act of 1973

This Act was designed to help facilitate the integration of people with disabilities into society (Hums 1991). The Act's purpose is "to develop and implement, through research, training, services and the guarantee of equal opportunity, comprehensive and coordinated programs of vocational rehabilitation and independent living" (Closen et al. 1989). The Act defines a disabled individual as "Any person who

1. has a physical or mental impairment that substantially limits one of such person's major life activities
2. has a record of such an impairment
3. is regarded as having such an impairment" (45 CFR 84.3(j)(1), 1997).

What are physical impairments and major life activities? The Act defines a physical impairment as:

Any physiological disorder or condition, cosmetic disfigurement, or anatomical loss affecting one or more of the following body systems: neurological; musculoskeletal; special sense organs; respiratory including speech organs; cardiovascular; reproductive; digestive; genito-urinary; hemic and lymphatic; skin; and endocrine; or any mental or psychological disorder, such as mental retardation, organic brain syndrome, emotional or mental illness, and specific learning disabilities. (45 CFR 84.3(j)(2)(i), 1997)

The Act delineates major life activities as "functions such as caring for one's self, performing manual tasks, walking, seeing, hearing, speaking, breathing, learning or working" (45 CFR 84.3(j)(2)(ii), 1997). In 1987, the Act was modified to clarify the policy with respect to people impaired by contagious conditions (Hums 1991).

In order to receive full protection under Section 504, individuals must prove not only that they are disabled but are otherwise qualified as defined by the act. The watershed case for examining whether people with contagious diseases are both disabled and otherwise qualified is *School Board of Nassau County, Florida v. Arline* ("*Arline*") (1987). Arline was discharged from her position as an elementary school teacher after she had three bouts of tuberculosis during a two-year period (MacFarlane 1989). To determine whether someone is otherwise qualified under the *Arline* standard, a person is entitled to the opportunity to have his or her condition evaluated in light of medical evidence. Also, any decision to exclude someone must be based on "reasonable medical judgments given the state of medical knowledge" (Mitten 1993). The court held that a person who creates a significant risk of communicating the disease to others is not otherwise qualified. In *Arline*, the court stated that risk should be assessed by

- the nature of the risk (how the disease is transmitted),
- the duration of the risk (how long is the carrier infectious),
- the severity of the risk (what the potential harm is to third parties), and
- the probability the disease will be transmitted and will cause varying degrees of harm.

Section 504 of the Rehabilitation Act of 1973 set the groundwork for protecting the rights of people with disabilities. The ADA, passed in 1990, expanded upon this base.

The Americans With Disabilities Act

Passed in the summer of 1990, the ADA has four purposes. First, it provides a clear and comprehensive national mandate for the elimination of discrimination against people with disabilities. Second, it provides a prohibition of discrimination against persons with disabilities. This prohibition is parallel in scope to the coverage afforded to persons discriminated against on the basis of race, sex, national origin, or religion. Third, the ADA provides clear, strong, consistent, enforceable standards addressing discrimination against people with disabilities. Fourth, the act invokes the sweep of congressional authority, including its power to enforce the fourteenth amendment, to regulate commerce, and to regulate interstate transportation. This allows the Act to address the major areas of discrimination faced day-to-day by people with disabilities (42 USC §12101(b), 1995)

The ADA contains sections about employment, public services, public accommodations, and services operated by private entities and telecommunications. This chapter will discuss the issues related to employment and public accommodations.

The Preface and Part I, Employment, §12102(2), define what is meant by a disability. A person is considered to have a disability if he or she

- has a physical or mental impairment that substantially limits one or more of the major life activities of such individual,
- has a record of such impairment, and
- is regarded as having such an impairment.

The ADA itself does not define major life activities. However, they are usually considered to be day-to-day activities like walking, talking, seeing, hearing, caring for oneself, breathing, sitting, standing, lifting, reaching, learning, working, reasoning, and remembering (Allen 1993). These activities are similar to those described by Section 504 of the Rehabilitation Act of 1973.

According to the United States Department of Justice (1996), HIV-positive persons, whether or not they have symptoms, have physical impairments that substantially limit one or more major life activities. Therefore, the law protects these individuals. In addition, the law protects those who are discriminated against because they are regarded as having AIDS. The ADA also protects those persons discriminated against because they have a known association or relationship with an HIV-positive individual (United States Department of Justice 1996).

Both the ADA and Section 504 of the Rehabilitation Act of 1973 help define the rights of people with disabilities and, specifically, people who are HIV positive. The next section discusses how this legislation and additional court cases address participation in sport by HIV-positive individuals.

Participation in Sport

Can HIV-positive individuals be forced to limit their participation in sport activities? To address this issue, one must first look at participation in sport by people with disabilities. Three sets of risk must be contemplated—risk to the infected individual, risk to competitors, and risk to the athlete's caregivers, such as trainers and team physicians. This section examines legal issues in three areas of participation—school-sponsored sports, health and fitness clubs, and recreational sports. The next section will discuss participation in professional sports since employment issues come into play for professional athletes.

School-Sponsored Sports

Athletes with disabilities have used three federal laws to secure participation in school-sponsored sports: the Rehabilitation Act of 1973, the ADA, and the Individuals with Disabilities Education Act (IDEA) (Wolohan 1996). According to Wolohan (1996), the Rehabilitation Act and the ADA are similar because they require an individual to establish the following points:

- that he or she is a disabled individual,
- that he or she is otherwise qualified for the activity,
- that he or she is being excluded solely by reason of the disability, and
- that the school or institution is a public or private entity for the ADA and receives financial assistance for §504.

The IDEA ensures all disabled children a free and appropriate public education that emphasizes special education and related services. Under the IDEA, a disabled student's formal individual education program (IEP) must ensure that a variety of educational, nonacademic, and extracurricular activities and services, including interscholastic athletics, are available to eligible students (Wolohan 1996).

In addition, some states have educational statutes prohibiting discrimination against elementary and high school athletes with disabilities (*Kampmeier v. Harris* 1978). Some courts have interpreted state human rights statutes as prohibiting unjustified discrimination against HIV-positive persons in places of public accommodation (*Minnesota v. Clausen* 1992). According to Mitten (1993), these state statutes may forbid excluding an HIV-positive athlete from participating in athletic events held in places of public accommodation, such as stadiums or arenas.

In a number of court cases, student-athletes with disabilities have won the opportunity to participate in sport. In *Wright v. Columbia University* (1981), the court granted the plaintiff, who had sight in only one eye, a temporary restraining order against the university, which had barred the plaintiff's participation in intercollegiate football. A student with one kidney was allowed to participate in interscholastic wrestling (*Poole v. South Plainfield Board of Education* 1980). In *Kampmeier v. Harris* (1978), a student who suffered from a congenital eye problem was allowed to participate under the condition that she wear protective eye gear. On the other hand, in a number of cases, student-athletes have been denied the opportunity to participate. A student who was blind in one eye was not allowed to play football. The court reasoned that damage to the remaining good eye could potentially leave the student blind (*Spitaleri v. Nyquist* 1973). In *Colombo v. Sewanhka Central School District* (1976), the court ruled that a severely hearing-impaired student was not allowed to play football, lacrosse, or soccer because the student would not be able to identify the direction from which sounds come. This inability would put him at an increased risk for injury.

Numerous court cases have dealt with athletes with disabilities and their opportunities to participate. However, no court cases to date have directly dealt with HIV-positive sport participants. In fact, only two early cases specifically mention HIV status and sport participation. One case of note, however, is *Doe v. Dolton Elementary School Dist. No. 148* (1988). In this case, a 12-year-old, HIV-positive boy was excluded from attending the school's regular education classes and extracurricular activities. Doe's parents, on his behalf, filed a motion for a preliminary injunction that would allow him to attend. This motion was successful. However, in an interesting twist, the court ordered the school district to follow a number of directives, one of which was that Doe not engage in any contact sports sponsored by the school in curricular and extracurricular activities. Although the court ordered this, it did not directly mention any specific medical reason given for excluding Doe from contact sports (Mitten 1993).

A second case, *Ray v. School District of DeSoto County* (1987), dealt with school attendance by three hemophiliac brothers who also had tested positive for HIV. Testimony from the boys' treating physician states, "The Ray boys are probably already aware that they must avoid contact sports in the school environment" (*Ray*, p. 1537). However, no additional information is given with the statement as to whether the physician was referring to their hemophilia or their HIV-positive status. While no court cases have involved allowing HIV-positive individuals to play sport, if one were brought, the courts would likely examine the risk of transmission based on current medical knowledge.

Health and Fitness Clubs

Clearly, the ADA covers access to sport facilities and programs for people with disabilities by its very definition of a place of public accommodation. A place of public accommodation means a facility operated by a private entity whose operations affect commerce and fall within a number of categories. Those categories, as specifically related to sport, include:

- a motion picture house, theater, concert hall, stadium, or other place of exhibition or entertainment;
- a park, zoo, amusement park, or other place of recreation;
- a gymnasium, health spa, bowling alley, golf course, or other place of exercise or recreation (42 USC §12181 (7), 1995).

Can a place of public accommodation exclude a person who is HIV positive because that person may be perceived to pose a direct threat to others? The answer to this question is invariably no since people with HIV/AIDS rarely, if ever, pose a direct threat in public accommodations. According to the ADA, a direct threat "means a significant risk to the health or safety of others that cannot be eliminated by reasonable accommodation" (42 USC §12111 (3), 1995).

According to the United States Department of Justice (1996):

> The determination that a person poses a direct threat to the health and safety of others may not be based on generalizations or stereotypes about the effects of a particular disability; it must be based on an individual assessment that considers the particular activity and the actual abilities and disabilities of the individual. The individual assessment must be based on reasonable judgment that relies on current medical evidence.

HIV-positive members of health and fitness clubs are entitled to the same use of facilities as any other members. HIV-positive members cannot be charged extra fees, banned from steam rooms or saunas, or be allowed to use the club facilities only during limited hours (United States Department of Justice 1996). According to the International Health, Racquet and Sportsclub Association (IHRSA), employees of health and fitness clubs may not refuse to provide services to people with HIV unless a medical professional determines the individual poses a legitimate risk of infection (International Health, Racquet and Sportsclub Association 1996). A club that terminates a member because that member has HIV or AIDS is asking to be sued. Once again, according to International Health, Racquet and Sportsclub Association (1996):

> First, before you even learn a member or staff person has AIDS, establish a policy in your club that only those with an absolute need to know are told that a person has AIDS. If you or any other member of your staff discusses a person's health status too freely, your club could be sued for invasion of privacy.

Under the ADA, the only time a health club or other place of public accommodation can exclude an individual with HIV or AIDS from their club is if that individual's participation would result in a direct threat to the health or safety of others. The determination of whether an employee or member poses a direct threat must be based on reasonable judgment that relies on *current medical evidence.* You should consult a health care professional if you feel someone with HIV or AIDS is a risk to others at your club, because this determination leaves you open to a discrimination suit.

Recreational Sports

The ADA directly references places of public accommodation that would be considered recreational facilities, such as gymnasiums or arenas. However, many other places of public accommodation may, through direct or indirect services, also provide opportunities for recreational sports. Stein (1993) suggests that recreation and leisure facilities, programs, and activities need to be interpreted in the broadest sense. This should include:

- camping and other outdoor activities, including those in wilderness areas, risk and nonrisk activities, and adventure and ropes courses;
- outings including hiking and picnics;

- physical activities, including physical fitness programs;
- playground and play area activities, including those involving equipment;
- sport and games, including both participant and spectator roles; and
- swimming and other aquatic activities.

The ADA contains language pertaining to specific wilderness access in federal wilderness areas for people with disabilities who use wheelchairs. According to 42 USC §12207c (1) (1995):

In general, Congress reaffirms that nothing in the Wilderness Act is to be construed as prohibiting use of a wheelchair in a wilderness area by an individual whose disability requires use of a wheelchair, and consistent with the Wilderness Act no agency is required to provide any form of special treatment or accommodation, or to construct any facilities or modify any conditions of lands within a wilderness area in order to facilitate such use.

The ADA does not contain specific language dealing with people who are HIV positive in the public recreational sport setting. It simply includes interpretations as to what is a place of public accommodation. This topic remains an area of future discussion for professionals in this field who may lead, for example, backpacking trips or rafting expeditions in which HIV-positive individuals may wish to participate (Gullion 1996).

Employment Issues for Professional Athletes

The next section will examine employment issues related to HIV status. It will also present a specific example of a professional athlete who may be HIV positive. Professional athletes pose a complex dilemma in terms of HIV infection. According to Webber (1995), professional athletes face two factors that put them at higher risk than others. First, professional athletes often have a very distinctive lifestyle. Being young, rich, and famous, they face a lifestyle full of temptations that could potentially lead them to promiscuous behavior. Webber (1995) therefore suggests that thinking that professional athletes have a higher-than-average chance of contracting HIV is not unreasonable. Second, due to the physical nature of the games these professional athletes play, blood is shed as a matter of course. Therefore, athletes have an increased possibility of coming into contact with another athlete's blood despite the fact that no documented cases of HIV transmission have occurred in a sport setting. A brief explanation of relevant sections from the employment provisions of the ADA follow. Although the example used in this section involves professional athletes, the same laws discussed here also cover front-office employees who may be HIV positive.

ADA Coverage

According to Title I, §12111 [sec. 101] (5)(A) of the ADA, the term employer means, "A person engaged in an industry affecting commerce who has 15 or more employees for each working day in each of 20 or more calendar weeks in the current or preceding calendar year, and any agent of such person." Professional sports organizations fit this description. As employees of sport organizations, professional athletes are covered by the employment provisions of the ADA.

Qualified Individuals With a Disability

According to Title I, §12111 [sec. 101], (8) of the ADA, a qualified individual with a disability means, "An individual who, with or without reasonable accommodation, can perform the essential functions of the employment position that such an individual holds or desires." In order to qualify, a person must still meet certain prerequisites for a position. For example, in *Pandazides v. Virginia Board of Education* (1992), a teacher who could not pass the required national teachers' examination could be considered unqualified for a teaching position. In *Sawhill v. Medical College of Pennsylvania* (1996), the plaintiff, a licensed clinical pathologist diagnosed with clinical depression, was told that his termination was because he did not fit into his department's future plans. He later discovered that his termination was related to his disability. The plaintiff alleged that this termination based on his disability violated the ADA. The Medical College's motion to dismiss was denied. A professional athlete, in order to be a qualified individual, would have to have the requisite skills necessary to be a professional athlete in his or her sport.

Reasonable Accommodation and Undue Hardship

Employers may need to make reasonable accommodations for workers who have a disability. Employers need not make a reasonable accommodation if an undue hardship would result. According to Title I, §12111 [sec. 101], (9) of the ADA, a reasonable accommodation may include:

- making existing facilities used by employees reasonably accessible to and usable by individuals with disabilities; and
- job restructuring; part-time or modified work schedules; reassignment to a vacant position; acquisition or modification of equipment or devices; appropriate adjustment or modifications of examinations, training materials, or policies; the provision of qualified readers or interpreters; and other similar accommodations for individuals with disabilities.

According to Title I, §12111 [sec. 101], (10)(A) of the ADA, an undue hardship is "an action requiring significant difficulty or expense, when considered in light of the factors set forth in subparagraph (B)". Determining whether an accommodation would impose an undue hardship takes into consideration the nature and cost of the accommodation needed, the overall financial resources of the covered entity, and the type of operation or operations of the covered entity. Even given these guidelines, whether or not an accommodation results in undue hardship is determined on a case-by-case basis.

The courts have interpreted what constitutes a reasonable accommodation and what constitutes an undue hardship differently in different cases. Some reasonable accommodations include allowing an employee to work at home who experiences pain while commuting (*Sargent v. Litton Systems* 1994) and eliminating heavy lifting and strenuous work (*Henchey v. Town of North Greenbush* 1993). At times, however, the courts have indicated that the requested accommodations were unreasonable or would have resulted in undue hardship. Reasonable accommodation does not require allowing an employee who has unpredictable violent outbursts to remain in the workplace (*Mazzarella v. U.S. Postal Service* 1993) or accommodating frequent or unpredictable absences *(Jackson v. Veteran's Administration* 1994).

For a professional athlete, reasonable accommodations could be made. For example, a team may have to change practice or training schedules or requirements for an HIV-positive player, change the number or length of road trips, or change the number of games in which he or she may play (Anderson 1995). This is all based on the assumption that the player is still well enough to play at the level of skill needed to compete successfully as a professional athlete. However, the athlete would not have to be accommodated if he or she placed an undue hardship on the team, as explained in the preceding section. Webber (1995) sums up the status of the HIV-positive professional athlete as follows:

A player who is HIV positive is considered "handicapped" and is protected from discrimination, except in limited cases for insurance coverage. Unless a "significant risk" or "BFOQ" (bona fide occupational qualification) can be established, which is extremely unlikely in these cases, an employer cannot override that protection, and must take reasonable steps to accommodate what risk there is. Other players cannot refuse to work with that player, as it is not objectively reasonable for those players to believe the situation is unsafe. Other players also cannot override that player's protection through contract in a collective agreement.

Confidentiality Issues

A major debate revolves around confidentiality. If an individual is HIV positive, who needs to know? Do team doctors and trainers need to know? Do student trainers, coaches, teammates, opponents, and companies whose products an athlete endorses need to know? Where is the line drawn as to who really needs to know? What about confidentiality for the individual who is HIV positive? Having a life-threatening disease places a person in a certain light in society. However, having a life-threatening and often misunderstood disease leads to a totally different perception of the infected individual. How is that person's reputation and ability to find employment affected? What about the disdain with which the infected individual will be treated by those who are seriously misinformed about HIV, AIDS, and in particular, how HIV is transmitted? What does the law say to people in sport about all of this?

Ever since the Supreme Court first recognized a constitutional right to privacy in *Griswold v. Connecticut*, ongoing debate has tried to define what is meant by confidentiality. The courts have sent mixed messages regarding the privacy of HIV/AIDS-related information. For example, in *Woods v. White*, the courts ruled that an inmate's right to privacy was violated when his HIV status was revealed to nonmedical prison personnel and other inmates. In *In re John Doe v. City of New York* (1994), an airline worker claimed his privacy rights were violated when settlement of a discrimination suit was made public. In that case, Judge Frank Altamari wrote, "Individuals who are infected with the HIV clearly possess a constitutionally protected right to privacy regarding their condition" (*In re John Doe*). However, at times, the courts have ruled just the opposite. A hospital's disclosure about the HIV status of a physician to colleagues and former patients did not violate Pennsylvania's HIV confidentiality law (*In re Milton S. Hershey Medical Center* 1991). Also, a federal district court ruled that a firefighter's privacy could be intruded upon by a mandatory HIV test because the city had an interest in insuring neither the public nor another firefighter would be exposed to HIV in "high-risk" situations (*Anonymous Firefighter v. City of Willoughby* 1991). The varying outcomes of HIV privacy cases indicate that the courts have not found or applied a consistent analysis (Doughty 1994).

Two aspects must be dealt with when discussing confidentiality—access (who is permitted to obtain information) and control (who determines who has access to information) (Doughty 1994). In the sport setting, do the team physician and trainers have access to information? Who decides who controls access to the information—an athletic director, the general manager, or the players' union?

The law considers an HIV-positive person as someone with a disability. As previously stated, that individual is therefore afforded all the protections and rights available to any otherwise qualified individual with a disability. However, with HIV and AIDS, the disability involves an infectious, life-threatening illness. Parallels can be drawn from how confidential information is handled for people with other life-threatening illnesses. Yet, distinct differences exist between AIDS and other life-threatening illnesses that make confidentiality all the more important. First, those initially affected by the disease were primarily members of socially marginalized or disadvantaged groups (Claussen 1993; Doughty 1994; Hums 1994). Second, as AIDS spread, so did widespread discrimination against those who actually had the disease, anyone thought to be associated with these socially marginalized groups, and caretakers for those who suffered from the disease (Dunlap 1989). Third, all-too-frequent careless disclosure of what was thought to be confidential information frightened people with the disease. They then lost trust in the very legal and medical institutions that were supposed to help them (Doughty 1994; Rennert 1991). Sport situations are often perceived differently due to the amount of physical activity involved between participants and those working with them. Yet, no case of HIV transmission has occurred in a sport setting.

The United States Olympic Sports Medicine Committee issued an updated report to all national governing bodies concerning transmission of infectious agents during athletic competition. This document addresses confidentiality as follows (Garl 1995):

The Americans With Disabilities Act has determined that infection with HIV/AIDS is a disability and those infected are protected by federal law. It provides for confidentiality of those infected and restricts access to information about patients' conditions. It also requires informed consent for testing and requires that anyone tested must understand that the test results will become part of their permanent medical record. The ADA also directs that the "Right to Know" about some person's condition applies only in situations where there is a risk of transmission. Because no transmissions have been reported in athletics, there is no basis for obtaining confidential medical information about HIV/AIDS status.

Sport organizations need to establish organizational policies for protecting the confidentiality of HIV information. These policies must take into account the rights of the infected individual as well as those working with that person. Several types of information should be included in such a confidentiality policy (Hums 1994; Rennert 1991):

- General principles—explain the importance of confidentiality to athletes and staff.
- Information covered by confidentiality policy—includes information about athletes' test results or treatment for HIV-related illnesses.
- Individuals subject to confidentiality policy—could include team physicians, athletic trainers, student trainers, coaches, or athletic counselors.
- Competency and informed consent for disclosure of HIV-related information—athletes would sign a consent form to disclose their HIV status to the appropriate organizational members.
- Intra-agency access to and disclosure of HIV-related information—addresses the question "Who needs to know?" within the organization, the most difficult question of all.
- Extra-agency disclosure of HIV-related information—designates an individual (such as the head athletic trainer) within the sport organization to be a contact person with any outside group to which the athlete has consented to disclose HIV-related information.
- Penalties for unauthorized disclosure—includes disciplinary actions the sport organization will follow if unauthorized disclosures occur.

A sound confidentiality policy needs to take into account three guidelines. First, it must consider information regarding the most current information about HIV transmission. Second, the individuals establishing the policy should seek advice from legal counsel so the policy properly follows all pertinent legal considerations related to confidentiality. Third, the policy must protect the dignity of the infected individual, as he or she now faces an uncertain future in terms of health and social acceptance.

Testing

Should mandatory HIV testing occur for athletes on the professional, college, interscholastic, Olympic, or Paralympic level? This controversy swirled with Greg Louganis' revelation that he had tested HIV positive at the time he struck his head on the diving board in the 1988 Olympic Games in Seoul, Korea. Only Louganis and his coach knew about his condition. The doctor who wore no gloves when he stitched up Louganis' head was unaware of Louganis' condition. Can HIV testing be legally mandated for athletes?

A number of sport organizations have issued statements or policies regarding HIV status and sport participation (Hums 1994). The following sport organizations have expressed opposition to mandatory testing of athletes for HIV infection: the National Football League (1992), National Hockey League (1991), National Collegiate Athletic Association (1992), National Federation of State High School Associations (Mitten 1993), and United States Olympic Sports Medicine Committee (Garl 1995). Several authors (Anderson 1995; Mitten 1993, 1994; Webber 1995) have addressed the issue of mandatory HIV testing in sport and have outlined a number of reasons why mandatory testing is not acceptable. According to Mitten (1993, 1994), no compelling justification exists for involuntary testing of all athletes given the medical consensus concerning the extremely low probability of HIV transmission during athletic competition. Also, Mitten (1993, 1994) asserts that testing is probably illegal. Webber (1995) writes that the idea of mandatory AIDS testing should be put to rest by implementing leaguewide bans on such procedures. On the other hand, Anderson (1995) suggests that leagues should attempt to undertake integrated, safety-minded, and educational mandatory HIV testing policies aimed at informing those infected of their status and the treatment available to them. Anderson (1995) also writes that leagues may consider including such testing in future collective bargaining discussions.

One particular exception to this is boxing. Ever since boxer Tommy Morrison announced his HIV-positive status, the boxing industry has started to look twice at mandatory testing. As of early 1996, the boxing commissions of at least nine states— Arizona, Georgia, Massachusetts, Nevada, New Mexico, New York, Oregon, Utah, and Washington—as well as of Puerto Rico require HIV testing (Massachusetts Boxing Commission 1996). Other states have indicated they will follow the trend. According to Skeeter McClure, the Massachusetts commission's chair,

> The decision is for the protection of the fighters, and the people who come in contact with the fighters, like the referees or physicians. . . . It's a contact sport where fluids, namely blood, are exchanged through clutching or gloves or other ways. It's in the best interest of everybody. (Massachusetts Boxing Commission 1996)

The World Boxing Council now requires all boxers in major fights to undergo HIV tests (WBC 1992). Look for this trend to continue. As of yet, no legal challenges have been made to mandatory testing in professional boxing.

Rights of the Individual Who Undergoes Testing

An individual usually has two choices for testing—anonymous testing or confidential testing. With anonymous testing, the person's name is never disclosed to anyone. Even the people doing the testing do not know the client's name. With confidential testing, often done at a doctor's office, local health department, or clinic, a person's name is recorded, but information about the test cannot be given to anyone without the client's consent. However, the results will be known to the client, the lab that did the testing, and the doctor's office. The test information becomes part of the client's records. With anonymous testing, a person's identity is never disclosed. With confidential testing, the person's name is attached to the results, thus increasing the risk of information about the person becoming known if the information is not properly secured (Georgia AIDS Information Line 1998). Numerical information about positive tests is provided to local health officials so the spread of the infection can be tracked. Thirty states require reporting of both AIDS and HIV-positive results with personal identifiers (such as names), while twenty states require reporting of only AIDS cases (United States Department of Health and Human Services—Centers for Disease Control and Prevention 1997).

Conclusion and Recommendations

Should HIV-positive athletes be allowed to participate in sport? Until medical science proves otherwise, only limited legal bases allow the exclusion of HIV-positive individuals from sport. Current medical knowledge concerning transmission of HIV and AIDS indicates that HIV cannot be transmitted in the sport setting. Therefore, unilateral banning of HIV-positive participants from sport is not needed.

Who should know about an athlete's HIV status? This question does not have definitive answers. It weaves the law together with a great number of considerations. The overriding fact, based on medical knowledge at this time, is that a documented case of HIV transmission has never occurred in sport. Therefore, the widespread broadcasting of an athlete's HIV status does not seem to have a legal basis. Rather, the prudent sport organization will develop and adhere to a legally and ethically sound confidentiality policy.

Obviously, the subject of HIV status and sport is a very complex matter, intertwining social, legal, ethical, economic, political, and educational considerations. Sport managers walk an uneasy tightrope involving HIV-positive status and sport. On one hand is the HIV-positive individual who wishes either to participate in sport or to work for a sport organization. On the other hand is the concern over the health and safety of the others with whom the HIV-positive individual interacts on a day-to-day basis on the playing field, in the gym, or in the office. While no known cases of HIV transmission have occurred in a sport setting, many misconceptions about HIV and how it is transmitted still persist. Sport managers need to know that people fall into three levels of understanding about AIDS and HIV infection. The first level consists of people who are educated about the disease. Sport managers need to incorporate the thoughts and ideas of these individuals to help sport organizations develop sound policies. The second level is made up of people who are not educated but can be. Here, the socially responsible sport organization can act as a leader in providing educational information to the public about HIV and AIDS so that these individuals will come to understand the illness. People in sport have a great amount of influence in society and can use their status to dispel fears and provide accurate information. The third group of people are those who refuse to be educated. Unfortunately, perhaps even sport organizations would have no influence over this particular group of individuals who will not listen to the facts from any source. This should not deter sport managers from continuing to provide proper information to the public.

Decisions concerning HIV-positive sport participants must be made not just following the letter of the law but considering the spirit of justice as well. Applying universal precautions to protect against disease transmission is one thing. Socially responsible sport managers must ask if they can apply universal precautions to one's human dignity as well.

References

Allen, J.G. (1993). *Complying With the ADA: A Small Business Guide to Hiring and Employing the Disabled.* New York: Wiley.

Americans With Disabilities Act of 1990, 42 U.S.C. §12101 *et seq.* (1995).

Anderson, P.M. (1995). Cautious defense: Should I be afraid to guard you? (Mandatory AIDS testing in professional team sports). *Marquette Sports Law Journal, 5* (2):279–315.

Anonymous Firefighter v. City of Willoughby, 779 F. Supp. 402 (N.D. Ohio, 1991).

Claussen, C.L. (1993). HIV positive athletes and the disclosure dilemma for athletic trainers. *Journal of Legal Aspects of Sport, 3* (2):25–34.

Closen, M.L., Herman, D.H., Horne, P.J., Isaacman, S.H., Jarvis, R.M., Leonard, A.S., Rivera, R., Scherzer, M., Scholtz, G.P., & Wojcik, M.E. (1989). *AIDS: Cases and Materials.* Houston, TX: John Marshall.

Colombo v. Sewanhka Central School District, 383 N.Y.S.2d 518 (N.Y. App. Div. 1976).

Doe v. Dolton Elementary School District No. 148, 694 F. Supp. 440 (N.D. Ill., 1988).

Doughty, R. (1994). The confidentiality of AIDS related information: Responding to the resurgence of aggressive public health interventions in the AIDS epidemic. *California Law Review, 82* (1):113–84.

Dunlap, M. (1989). AIDS and discrimination in the United States: Reflections on the nature of prejudice in a virus. *Villanova Law Review, 34* (5):909.

Garl, T. (1995). *Transmission of Infectious Agents During Athletic Competition.* Colorado Springs: United States Olympic Committee.

Georgia AIDS Information Line (1998, May 15). Personal communication.

Griswold v. Connecticut, 381 U.S. 479, 85 S. Ct. 1678 (1965).

Gullion, L. (1996, November 14). Personal communication.

Henchey v. Town of North Greenbush, 831 F. Supp. 960 (N.D. N.Y., 1993).

Hums, M.A. (1991). AIDS and sports participants: Legal and ethical considerations for school sports programs. *Journal of Legal Aspects of Sport, 1* (1):22–35.

Hums, M.A. (1994). AIDS in the sports arena: After Magic Johnson, where do we go from here? *Journal of Legal Aspects of Sport, 4* (1):59–65.

International Health, Racquet and Sportsclub Association (IHRSA). (1996). *Acquired Immune Deficiency Syndrome (AIDS): An IHRSA Briefing Paper.* Boston: International Health, Racquet and Sportsclub Association.

In re John Doe v. City of New York, 1994 WL 24213 825 F. Supp 36 (SDNY, 1994).
In re Milton S. Hershey Medical Center, 595 A.2d 1290 (Pa Super., 1991).
Jackson v. Veteran's Administration, 22 F.3d 277 (11th Cir. 1994).
Kampmeier v. Harris, 411 N.Y.S.2d 744 (N.Y. App. Div. 1978).
MacFarlane, M.A. (1989). Equal opportunities: Protecting the rights of AIDS-linked children in the classroom. *American Journal of Law and Medicine, 14* (4):377–430.
Massachusetts Boxing Commission Institutes Mandatory HIV Testing. (1996). Retrieved October 15, 1998 from the World Wide Web: **http://www3.nando. net/newsroom/ap/oth/1996/oth/box/feat/archive/022796/box61293. html**
Mazzarella v. U.S. Postal Service, 849 F. Supp. 89 (D. Mass., 1993).
Minnesota v. Clausen, 491 N.W.2d 662 (Minn. Ct. App. 1992).
Mitten, M.J. (1993). AIDS and athletics. *Seton Hall Journal of Sport Law, 3* (1):5–40.
Mitten, M.J. (1994). HIV-positive athletes: When medicine meets the law. *The Physician and Sportsmedicine, 22* (10):63–64, 67–68.
National Collegiate Athletic Association. (1992). *1992 NCAA Sports Medicine Handbook.* Overland Park, KS: National Collegiate Athletic Association.
National Football League. (1992). *National Football League HIV/AIDS Related Policies.* New York: National Football League.
National Hockey League. (1991). Memo provided by the National Hockey League office.
Pandazides v. Virginia Board of Education, 804 F. Supp. 794 (E.D. Va., 1992).
Poole v. South Plainfield Board of Education, 490 F. Supp. 948 (D. N.J., 1980).
Ray v. School District of DeSoto County, 666 F. Supp. 1524 (M.D. Fla., 1987).
Rehabilitation Act of 1973, 29 U.S.C. §§ 701–796i. (1996).
Rennert, S. (1991). AIDS/HIV and confidentiality: Model policy and procedures. *Kansas Law Review, 39* (3):653–737.
Sargent v. Litton Systems, 841 F. Supp. 956 (N.D. Cal., 1994).
Sawhill v. Medical College of Pennsylvania, 1996 U.S. Dist. LEXIS 4097 (E.D. Pa., 1996).
School Board of Nassau County, Florida v. Arline ("Arline"), 480 U.S. 273 (1987).
Spitaleri v. Nyquist, 345 N.Y.S. 2d 878 (N.Y. App. Div. 1973).
Stein, J. (1993). The Americans With Disabilities Act: Implications for recreation and leisure. In S.J. Grosse & D. Thompson (Eds.), *Leisure Opportunities for Individuals with Disabilities: Legal Issues* (pp. 1–11). Reston, VA: American Alliance for Health, Physical Education, Recreation and Dance.
United States Department of Health and Human Services—Centers for Disease Control and Prevention. (1997). *HIV/AIDS Surveillance Report.* Atlanta, GA: Centers for Disease Control and Prevention.
United States Department of Justice. (1996). *Questions and Answers: The Americans With Disabilities Act and Persons with HIV/AIDS.* Retrieved July 1, 1997 from the World Wide Web: **gopher://justice.2.usdoj.gov: 70/00/crt/ada/ hivqanda.txt**
WBC sets HIV tests for fights. (1992, November 14). *New York Times*, p. 31.
Webber, D.M. (1995). When the "Magic" rubs off: The legal implications of AIDS in professional sports. *Sports Lawyers Journal, 2* (1):1–24.

Wolohan, J. (1996). Why high school athletic associations should conduct case by case reviews before barring the disabled athlete. *For the Record, 7* (1):5, 7.
Woods v. White, 689 F.Supp. 874 (N.D. Wi., 1988).
Wright v. Columbia University, 520 F. Supp. 789 (E.D. Pa., 1981).

Conclusion and Recommendations

Gopal Sankaran, Karin A. E. Volkwein, and Dale R. Bonsall
West Chester University of Pennsylvania

The preceding chapters have outlined and discussed the challenges and opportunities associated with human immunodeficiency virus (HIV) infection and the resultant acquired immunodeficiency syndrome (AIDS) as they pertain to sport. A cure or a vaccine to prevent an individual from acquiring HIV is not yet available. Fortunately, the risk of HIV transmission in sport settings is infinitesimally small. Proper use of universal precautions for blood-borne pathogens provide proven, effective methods of prevention against contracting HIV. Additionally, both amateur and professional athletes must pay due attention to the risk of acquiring HIV infection outside the sport arena and take adequate precautions to protect themselves from this virus. Thus, individuals have to take measures to protect themselves in every life setting, including sport.

Attitudes are shaped early in the life of an individual. The notion of invincibility established during early adolescence is carried through late adolescence and young adulthood, when people are most likely to be involved in competitive sports. This misconception often prevents these individuals from thinking rationally and readily accepting proven strategies of risk-reduction measures to prevent both contraction and transmission of HIV. This scenario poses an even greater challenge for parents, athletic trainers, coaches, game officials, sport administrators, and health care providers, who care and guide these young individuals. These professionals must become more educated about HIV and its impact. They should clarify their values to be nonjudgmental in their support of HIV-positive individuals. These professionals should also learn to make effective use of appropriate resources to combat the ignorance and stigma associated with AIDS.

HIV-negative athletes and those who consider themselves to be not infected with HIV may find mandatory testing of all athletes for HIV infection intuitively appealing. However, mandatory testing is fraught with problems. These include infringement on the rights of those who are already infected with the virus, stigmatization, social ostracism, and the inability to detect those in the window period—who may be infected with HIV but have a false negative HIV antibody test. Universal precautions, when applied accurately and consistently, provide a reliable protection against HIV transmission in sport settings. So far, contraction of HIV among athletes (both professionals and amateurs) has occurred solely due to the practice of risky behaviors outside the sporting arenas. The possibility of HIV transmission in sport settings is often raised, especially when the media focus on a celebrity athlete who has been infected with HIV. Such teachable moments should be seized upon to allow for open, honest discussion about the known modes of HIV transmission. These opportunities could help dispel myths and misconceptions surrounding the infection and its impact. Education is the key to check the spread of HIV and, therefore, has to be provided both on and off the field. This is not an easy task, but neither is it an impossible one.

The rights to privacy and confidentiality of those who have contracted HIV need to be respected. At the same time, the rights of uninfected individuals in their need to be protected from HIV should be considered. Upholding the rights of those infected with and those not infected with HIV often creates tension. Policies and procedures need to be in place to balance the rights of the individuals and the obligations of the institutions involved in sport. Sport institutions, organizations, and clubs (both domestic and international) need to develop policies that are humanistic, ethical, and based on available current scientific evidence. Policies based on emotional feelings alone are bound to create rift in sport. Judicious administration of policies through a set of standardized guidelines is necessary. Several domestic and international sports organizations have already taken a lead in this matter. However, the differences in domestic and international policies still need to be reconciled. These differences are particularly evident in contact sports, such as wrestling.

Given the effectiveness of universal precautions, (when properly applied), mandatory testing of athletes for HIV infection is not needed. No one really benefits by knowing the HIV status of the fellow athlete or opponent. Exclusion of an HIV-positive athlete from competition does not enhance sport. It disenfranchises the HIV-positive athlete and annuls the contribution that the person could continue to make to sport.

An athlete with HIV can continue to contribute to sport and, in time, can benefit physically, socially, and emotionally from such participation. A number of examples abound, and the text has discussed these. In the foreseeable future, AIDS may well become a chronic disease. Society will witness a greater recognition of the impact of the disease on athletes, coaches, athletic trainers, sport personalities, and others involved with sport. The United States alone has about 650,000–900,000 persons infected with HIV. Almost half of these individuals do not know that they are infected with HIV. Many of the infected are likely to be athletes—amateurs and professionals. The authors reiterate that HIV-positive individuals *do not* pose an additional threat to those who are free of the HIV infection *if* universal precautions against blood-borne pathogens are taken in the sport arena. These precautions have to be observed at all times and should not be based on a mythical ability to predict which athlete is possibly infected and which athlete is not. This eliminates one possible means of discrimination and achieves effective protection of uninfected persons. The authors hope that discrimination against HIV-infected individuals will be eliminated. Educating people about the actual modes of HIV transmission and the ways they could avoid contracting or transmitting HIV could reduce this discrimination.

The authors do not recommend mandatory testing for all athletes (amateurs or professionals). However, they do strongly advocate that those who suspect they may be infected with HIV should undergo voluntary testing with pretest and posttest counseling. This is critical. Early diagnosis and prompt initiation of treatment is vital for increasing the quality and length of one's life. These advantages are lost when HIV-positive individuals postpone or never undertake testing for HIV infection. The responsibility for getting tested rests with the individual. All those who care for and guide these individuals need to support the athletes irrespective of the test results. Persons who develop policies and procedures for sport organizations and those who are responsible for implementing them have to be nonjudgmental of the HIV-infected athletes and sensitive to their rights.

Society must deal with HIV infection and the resultant AIDS on a scientific basis rather than on an emotional one, which is often laced with biases and misplaced beliefs. Such a task is not easy. Each person has the responsibility to educate himself or herself about the current developments related to HIV/AIDS and be able to take an objective position in developing policies and procedures for the world of sport. This can be achieved only through united, well-coordinated, educational efforts. The time to take a courageous step in this direction is now. The authors hope that this text has aided in this process.

Glossary

Acquired immunodeficiency syndrome (AIDS): A manifestation of infection with the human immunodeficiency virus (HIV) characterized by the presence of one or more diseases as defined by the Centers for Disease Control and Prevention (CDC). These diseases occur following depression of an individual's immune system function. The affected person becomes susceptible to unusual infections and malignancies.

Aerosolized pentamidine: A drug used for *Pneumocystis carinii* pneumonia (PCP) prophylaxis that is dispersed through a nebulizer in a mist. When inhaled, it goes directly into the lungs.

Airborne transmission: Process by which an infectious agent passes through the air to infect susceptible individuals by droplet infection (for example, sneezing and coughing).

Americans with Disabilities Act: (Public Law 101-336) Passed in July 1990, this legislation establishes equal opportunity for persons with disabilities regarding employment, public accommodation, transportation, state and local government services, and telecommunications.

Antibodies: Proteins in the blood or secretory fluids that tag and help remove or neutralize bacteria, viruses, and other harmful toxins. Antibodies are members of a class of proteins known as immunoglobulins, which are produced and secreted by B-lymphocytes in response to stimulation by antigens.

Antigen: A substance, usually protein or polysaccharide in composition, that stimulates a response from the immune system resulting in the production of specific antibodies.

Antiretroviral drug: A drug that reduces the replication rate of HIV and is used to treat HIV-infected persons. Common ones include zidovudine, didanosine, and zalcitabine.

Asymptomatic HIV infection: An early stage of HIV infection in which the person has no physical symptoms.

ß$_2$-microglobulin: A type of microglobulin. Microglobulins are any globulin or fragment of a globulin of low-molecular weight. It is a serum marker of the inflammatory response that may be elevated in persons with progressive HIV disease.

B-lymphocyte: Also called B-cell. A white blood cell that plays an important role in the human immune system. It is associated with humoral immunity. It secretes antibodies (soluble proteins) specific to the antigen eliciting the response.

Bias: Any action at any stage of a study that leads to systematic error in study results.

Bioassay: The process of determining the strength of a compound by its effect upon microorganisms, animals, or tissues. Usually a reference standard is used in the process.

Body fluids: The various liquids found in the human body. Of these fluids, only blood, semen, vaginal secretions, and breast milk have been found to contain concentrations of HIV high enough to infect another person. Saliva, sweat, tears, and urine have not been shown to transmit HIV.

Casual contact: In the context of HIV infection and AIDS, refers to nonintimate behaviors such as hugging, holding hands, playing, eating, and working together. These activities do not transmit HIV.

CD (cluster designation): Cell surface protein molecules present on the surface of lymphocytes and other cells in humans. These surface protein molecules serve as attachment sites for HIV. They also help to classify different types of lymphocytes.

CD4+ cell count (T4 count): A surrogate marker of immunodeficiency; the number of CD4+ (T4-helper) cells. As an HIV-positive individual's CD4+ cells decline, the risk of developing opportunistic infections increases. The trend of several consecutive CD4+ counts is more important than any one measurement.

CD4+ percentage: The number of CD4+ cells in relation to the total number of lymphocytes. As HIV infection progresses, the percentage of CD4+ cells decreases.

CD8+ cell count (T8 count): The number of CD8+ cells in the body. CD8+ cells are a type of leukocytes or white blood cells in the body. CD8+ cells are also known as T-suppressor cells. They are capable of suppressing the activity of other immune cells or processes.

CD45RA+ and CD45RO+ cell populations: CD4+ T-lymphocytes are broadly categorized into naive and memory populations. This categorization is based on expression of different forms of CD45+ (leukocyte common antigen) found on the cell surface. CD45RA+ (the high-molecular weight CD45+ isoform) is a marker of the naive subset of T-lymphocytes. The CD45RO+ (the low-molecular weight isoform) is a marker of the reciprocal memory subset of T-lymphocytes. In the literature, the CD45RA+ is often indicated as CD4+45RA+ and the CD45RO+ cell as CD4+45RO+.

CD56+ cell: A subtype of natural killer (NK) cells. See *Natural killer cell.*

Cell-mediated immunity (CMI): A type of immune response in humans associated with cellular components such as T-lymphocytes. See also *Humoral immunity.*

Centers for Disease Control and Prevention (CDC): Federal agency responsible for monitoring the HIV/AIDS epidemic and carrying out efforts to prevent and control the spread of HIV.

Central nervous system (CNS): The brain, spinal cord, and its coverings (meninges).

Cohort: A group of individuals sharing a demographic or clinical characteristic.

Condom: A sheath used to cover the penis during sexual intercourse to prevent pregnancy and transmission of sexually transmissible infections, including HIV.

Confidentiality: The right inherent in the contract between the health care provider and patient that ensures that information about the patient's medical conditions will be released to a third party only after explicit permission is obtained from the patient or guardian.

Constitutional symptoms: Symptoms or complaints related to the whole human body or the functional habit of the body (such as those affecting physiological processes). Constitutional symptoms include fever, body aches, general weakness, and so on. These differ from local symptoms such as localized pain or swelling.

Cubic millimeter: Millimeter refers to one-thousandth of a meter. Cubic millimeter is denoted as mm³.

Cytotoxic T-cell: Also known as lymphokine-activated killer (LAK) cell. The helper T-cells (or CD4+ cells) release lymphokines that stimulate other T-lymphocytes known as the cytotoxic T-cells. These lymphocytes then migrate from the lymph nodes to the circulatory system to the site of the microbe-infected cells and then destroy them.

DNA: Deoxyribonucleic acid. A nucleic acid containing deoxyribose as the sugar component. It is the autoreproducing component of chromosomes and of many viruses. It is the repository of hereditary characteristics. See *RNA*.

Diagnosis: Determination of the nature of a disease.

Early HIV infection: The stage of HIV infection during which no major physical health symptoms are yet present, though psychological symptoms may be present.

Enzyme-linked immunosorbent assay (ELISA): The most common assay for HIV antibodies. It is used to screen donated blood and is usually the first clinical screening test used to detect HIV infection. A positive ELISA test result should be confirmed with a western blot or an immunofluorescent assay test to diagnose HIV infection conclusively.

Epidemic: An outbreak of contagious disease, such as HIV infection, that spreads rapidly within a population.

Epidemiology: The study of the distribution and determinants of disease frequency in a population.

Etiology: The study of the causes of disease.

Food and Drug Administration (FDA): Federal agency responsible for approving new pharmaceutical products and medical devices and for monitoring drug performance following approval.

Genome: All of the chromosomes found in a cell. Chromosomes carry the genes, the functional unit of heredity.

gp: Refers to glycoprotein, a protein molecule with one or more carbohydrate groups.

gp41, gp120, gp160: Types of glycoproteins; the numbers indicate their molecular weight.

Granuloma: Inflammatory lesions that are usually nodular, firm, and persistent with a special cellular content (mononuclear phagocytes that are compactly grouped).

HIV: Human immunodeficiency virus.

HIV antibody (HIV Ab): The antibody to HIV, which usually appears within six weeks after infection. Antibody testing early in the infection process may not produce accurate results since some recently infected people have not yet begun producing antibodies. Therefore, some individuals test negative even though they are infected. Thus, in some situations, a single negative antibody test result does not guarantee that a person is free from infection. The change from HIV-negative to HIV-positive status is called seroconversion.

HIV counseling: Information provided to an individual before and after HIV testing (pretest and posttest counseling) regarding the implications and impact of testing, HIV infection care, and prevention of HIV transmission.

HIV disease: The entire natural history of infection with human immunodeficiency virus from the time of infection to the gradual progression of the disease, development of clinical AIDS, resultant complications, and ensuing death.

HIV infected: Infected with the human immunodeficiency virus, with or without evidence of illness.

HIV negative: Not infected with HIV, as determined by a negative test for antibody to HIV or for the presence of the virus.

HIV positive: Infected with HIV, as determined by a positive test for antibody to HIV or for the presence of the virus.

Human immunodeficiency virus (HIV): The organism isolated and recognized as the causal agent of AIDS. It infects and destroys a class of lymphocytes, CD4+ cells, thereby causing progressive damage to the immune system. Two types of HIV are known. HIV-1 is the most common form in the United States. HIV-2 causes a milder immune suppression and is found primarily in Africa.

Humoral immunity: A type of immunologic response that occurs in the body fluids (humors) and is orchestrated by B-lymphocytes. The effect is mediated through the production of immunoglobulins. See *Immunoglobulins.*

Immune system: The mechanism of the body that recognizes foreign agents or substances, neutralizes them, and recalls the response later when confronted with the same challenge.

Immunity: Natural or acquired resistance to a specific disease. Immunity may be partial or complete, long lasting or temporary.

Immunocompromised: Describes the condition that exists when the body's immune system defenses are lowered and the ability to resist infections and tumors weakens.

Immunodeficiency: A breakdown or an inability of certain parts of the immune system to function. This renders a person susceptible to certain diseases that he or she ordinarily would not develop.

Immunoglobulins (Ig): Proteins produced by plasma cells derived from B-lymphocytes and found in the blood and other body tissues. Increased levels of two types of immunoglobulins, immunoglobulin A (IgA) and immunoglobulin G (IgG), are usually seen in patients with HIV infection and are related to the HIV-induced activation of B-lymphocytes. IgA is found in high concentrations in mucous membranes and in secretions such as saliva. It does not cross the placenta. IgG is found in the serum and does cross the placenta.

Immunopathogenesis: The mechanisms that result in disease of the immune system.

Incubation period: The interval between initial infection and appearance of the first symptom or sign of disease.

Informed consent: Process by which an individual voluntarily consents to diagnostic testing and the release of information (disclosure) after appropriate counseling.

Interleukin: A class of lymphokines important for lymphocyte proliferation. Several types, such as interleukin-1 (IL-1) and interleukin-2 (IL-2), are known. See *Lymphokine.*

In vitro: Testing and experiments conducted in a laboratory setting.

In vivo: Testing and experiments conducted in animals or humans.

Kaposi's sarcoma (KS): A painless tumor of the wall of blood vessels or the lymphatic system that usually appears on the skin as pink to purple spots. It may also occur internally, independent of skin lesions.

Leukocyte: A white blood cell.

Lymphocyte: A type of white blood cell in the human body. The most prominent cell type in the immune system. B-lymphocytes are one of the two major classes of lymphocytes. During infections, these cells are transformed into plasma cells that produce antibodies specific to the invading pathogen. This transformation occurs through interactions with various types of T-lymphocytes and other components of the immune system. T-lymphocytes are derived from the thymus and participate in a variety of cell-mediated immune reactions. Three fundamentally different types of T-lymphoytes exist: helper, killer, and suppressor.

Lymphokine: A generic term for soluble protein mediators released by sensitized lymphocytes on contact with specific antigens. They play a role in cell-mediated immunity.

Lymphokine-activated killer (LAK) cell: See *Cytotoxic T-cell.*

Lymphoma: Usually solid, well-defined, cancerous growth of lymph and reticuloendothelial tissues.

Macrophage: A special type of large, amoeboid, white blood cell capable of phagocytosis. In other words, it engulfs and destroys invading microorganisms. See *Phagocyte.*

Mandatory reporting: System under which a health care provider is required by law to inform health authorities when a specified illness is diagnosed. Mandatory reporting is required for AIDS in all 50 states. The Centers for Disease Control and Prevention has proposed that the requirement be extended for HIV infection.

Microbe: A microorganism, especially one that is capable of causing disease.

Microliter: A measure equivalent to one-millionth of a liter (μl).

Mitogen: A substance that stimulates cell division and lymphocyte transformation.

Monocyte: A type of leukocyte that destroys invading microorganisms by phagocytosis.

Myalgia: Pain in muscle tissue.

Myopathy: Inflammation of muscle tissue due to infection or adverse reaction to a medication.

Natural killer (NK) cell: This lymphocyte is less specialized than the cytotoxic T-cell (also known as lymphokine-activated killer (LAK) cell) and is apparently the primary mechanism for defense by the immune system against tumor cells. See also *Cytotoxic T-cell.*

Neuropathy: An abnormal, degenerative, or inflammatory condition of the peripheral nervous system.

Neutrophil: A type of mature white blood cell. It has a nucleus with three to five lobes connected by thin threads of chromatin. It has very fine granules present in the cytoplasm. Also known as polymorphonuclear leukocyte (PMNL).

Opportunistic infections (OIs): Illnesses caused by organisms that do not usually cause disease in a person with a healthy immune system. When an individual's immune system is compromised, such organisms may cause serious, even life-threatening illness.

p24 antigen test (p24 antigen capture assay): Laboratory test that measures p24, the protein found in the viral core of HIV. This test can sometimes detect HIV infection before seroconversion. p24 is consistently present in only about 25% of HIV-infected persons. Persistent high p24 antigen levels in blood have been associated with an increased risk of progression to AIDS in HIV-infected individuals.

Pandemic: An epidemic that involves many countries or regions of the world (that is, a worldwide epidemic).

Parenteral: Intravenous or intramuscular administration of substances such as therapeutic drugs or nutritive solutions.

Pathogenesis: Includes identifying the mode of origin, the cellular events and reactions, and other changes occurring in the body during the development of a disease.

Pentamidine: A drug used for PCP prophylaxis and treatment.

Perinatal transmission: Transmission of HIV from mother to infant by blood or body fluids. May occur in utero, at the time of delivery, and by breastfeeding.

Phagocyte: Any cell capable of ingesting particulate matter and microorganisms. Types of phagocytes include polymorphonuclear leukocytes, macrophages, and monocytes.

***Pneumocystis carinii* pneumonia (PCP):** Form of pneumonia seen in persons with an impaired immune system, such as those who are HIV infected. PCP is the leading cause of death in patients with AIDS. It is caused by the opportunistic pathogen, *Pneumocystis carinii,* which can infect the eyes, skin, spleen, liver, heart, as well as the lungs.

Polymerase chain reaction (PCR): A laboratory technique employing molecular biology technology. It can identify the nucleic acid sequence of HIV in the cells of an infected individual. This technique is sensitive and can detect a single copy of viral DNA in 1 cell out of 10,000. It is useful for early detection of perinatally infected infants and monitoring patients in clinical trials.

Primary care provider: A health care provider (for example, a physician, physician's assistant, or nurse practitioner) who offers and coordinates comprehensive patient care.

Prognosis: A prediction of the probable course and outcome of a disease in a person.

Prophylaxis: Intervention intended to preserve health and prevent the initial occurrence of a disease (primary prophylaxis) or to prevent the recurrence of a disease (secondary prophylaxis).

Protease inhibitors: The human immunodeficiency virus (HIV) has an enzyme, protease, that cleaves polyproteins into functional protein components during the late stages of HIV infection. When this cleavage is blocked, then an immature virus results, which is not capable of infecting new cells in the body. Protease inhibitors lead to competitive inhibition of the HIV protease by being complementary to the active site of the enzyme. Examples of this group of newer drugs include Saquinavir, Ritonavir, Indinavir, and Nelfinavir.

Reverse transcriptase: The enzyme present in HIV that converts viral RNA to DNA. This initiates the process that leads to the synthesis of viral proteins in an infected individual.

Risk reduction: Process by which an individual changes behavior so as to decrease the likelihood of acquiring an infection.

RNA: Ribonucleic acid. A nucleic acid with ribose as the sugar component. It is present in all living cells and controls cellular protein synthesis. It replaces deoxyribonucleic acid as a carrier of genetic codes in some viruses. See *DNA.*

Safe sex: In the context of HIV infection, sexual activity conducted in such a way that the risk of transmission or acquisition of the infection decreases (for example, having a single sexual partner who is not infected with HIV).

Safer sex: Sexual activity conducted in such a way that transmission of HIV infection is minimized by reducing the exchange of body fluids (for example, consistent use of condoms and avoiding unprotected sexual intercourse).

Sarcoidosis: A generalized (systematic) granulomatous condition of unknown cause. Involves lungs, lymph nodes, spleen, liver and other organs of the body. *See granuloma.*

Sensitivity: The ability of a test to identify correctly an individual who is infected.

Seroconversion: The process by which a person's antibody status changes from negative to positive.

Serological test: Any of a number of tests performed on the clear, liquid portion of the blood (serum). Often refers to a test that determines the presence of antibodies to antigens such as viruses.

Seronegative: Having a negative test for antibodies to a substance or organism, such as HIV.

Seropositive: Having a positive test for antibodies to a substance or organism, such as HIV.

Side effect: Action or effect of a drug other than that desired. The term usually refers to undesired or negative effects (for example, drug toxicity).

Sign: An indication of a disease or disorder observed by the health care provider.

Specificity: The ability of a test to identify correctly an individual who is not infected.

Symptom: Any perceptible, subjective change in the body or its functions that indicates disease or phases of disease, as reported by the patient.

Syndrome: A group of symptoms and diseases that together are characteristic of a specific condition.

T-lymphocyte: Also called T-cell. It is an important component of the human immune system and is associated with cell-mediated immunity. Different types exist such as helper, suppressor, or cytotoxic. This cell often is the host cell for the human immunodeficiency virus (HIV).

T-4 lymphocyte: Also called T-4 cell, T- helper cell, CD4+ lymphocyte, or CD4+ cell.

T-8 lymphocyte: Also called T-8 cell, T-suppressor cell, CD8+ lymphocyte, or CD8+ cell.

Thrush: An infection of the oral mucous membrane by *Candida albicans,* a fungus. It is usually seen as white patches on a red base on the inner cheeks. It can, however, occur anywhere in the mouth.

Trimethoprim-sulfamethoxazole (TMP-SMX): A first-line combination drug for PCP prophylaxis and treatment.

Universal precautions: A set of recommendations from the Centers for Disease Control and Prevention (CDC) to protect those who come in contact with body fluids that have the potential to transmit HIV. The universal blood and other body fluid precautions apply to semen, vaginal secretions, cerebrospinal fluid (CSF), and fluids from peritoneal, pleural, and pericardial cavities. Universal precautions are not applicable to saliva, sputum, sweat, feces, urine, vomitus, and breast milk, as the amount of HIV is rather low in them.

Vaccine: A substance that contains antigenic components of an infectious organism. Vaccines stimulate an immune response and may protect or modify subsequent infection by that organism.

Viral load/burden: The concentration of virus present in the body. This refers to the large number of HIV-infected cells in the body. The number of these cells may range from 10^{11} to 10^{12} in HIV-infected persons. HIV RNA levels, p24 antigen levels, and quantitative HIV culture measure the activity of this viral burden.

Viremia: Indicates the presence of viruses in the blood.

Virion: A complete viral particle found outside the cell. It is comprised of the nucleoid (genetic material) and the capsid (the protective protein shell). It is capable of infecting a living cell.

Virus: A class of infectious agents, which are very small in size, and do not contain the biochemical mechanisms for their own replication. They use the biochemical mechanisms of a host cell to synthesize and then assemble their various components.

$\dot{V}O_2$max: The maximum oxygen consumption, usually expressed as a volume of oxygen consumed per minute. It indicates maximal exercise power and is used to quantitate exercise rate among individuals.

Western blot (WB): A test to identify the presence of antibodies to multiple antigens of HIV; used to confirm HIV infection following a positive ELISA test. The WB displays antibodies to specific HIV viral proteins in a separate, well-defined band.

White blood cells (WBC): Cells that direct the normal immune system in a healthy adult. They consist of two classes of cells. The first, lymphocytes, respond to specific invading foreign organisms. The other class (macrophages, eosinophils, natural killer cells, and mast cells) nonspecifically attack invading foreign organisms.

References

El-Sadr, W., Oleske, J. M., Agins, B. D., Bauman, K. A., Brosgart, C. L., Brown, G. M., Geaga, J. V., Greenspan, D., Hein, K., Holzemer, W. L., Jackson, R. E., Lindsay, M. K., Makadon, H. J., Moon, M. W., Rappoport, C. A., Scott, G., Shervington, W. W., Shulman, L. C. & Wolfsy, C. B. (1994). *Evaluation and Management of Early HIV Infection. Clinical Practice Guideline No. 7.* (AHCPR Publication No. 94-0572.) Rockville, MD: U.S. Department of Health and Human Services, Public Health Service, Agency for Health Care Policy and Research.

Guide to Resources for HIV/AIDS

National Organizations

Advocates for Youth
1025 Vermont Avenue, NW, Suite 200
Washington, DC 20005
202-347-5700 (Voice)
202-347-2243 (Fax)

American Academy of Pediatrics (AAP)
141 North West Point Boulevard
PO Box 927
Elk Grove Village, IL 60009
847-228-5005

American Alliance for Health, Physical Education, Recreation and Dance
(AAHPERD)
1900 Association Drive
Reston, VA 22091
703-476-3400

The American Foundation for AIDS Research (AMFAR)
733 3rd Avenue, 12th Floor
New York, NY 10017
212-682-7440

American Medical Society for Sports Medicine (AMSSM)
7611 Elmwood Avenue, Suite 203
Middleton, WI 53562

American Orthopedic Society for Sports Medicine (AOSSM)
6300 North River Road, Suite 200
Rosemont, IL 60018
847-292-4900

American Public Health Association (APHA)
1015 15th Street, NW
Washington, DC 20005
202-789-5600

American Red Cross National Headquarters
8111 Gatehouse Road
Falls Church, VA 22042
202-737-8300

Gay Men's Health Crisis (GMHC)
119 West 24th Street
New York, NY 10011
212-367-1000 (Voice)
212-367-1220 (Fax)

National AIDS Information Clearinghouse
PO Box 6003
Rockville, MD 20850
301-762-5111 (Fax)
Reference Specialist
800-458-5231
Publications Orders
800-342-AIDS—24-hour AIDS hotline

National Association of People With AIDS (NAPWA)
1413 K Street, NW
Washington, DC 20005
202-898-0414

National Collegiate Athletic Association (NCAA)
6201 College Boulevard
Overland Park, KS 66211-2422
913-339-1906

National Federation of State High School Associations (NFSHSA)
PO Box 20626
Kansas City, MO 64195-0626
816-464-5400

National Minority AIDS Council
1931 13th Street, NW
Washington, DC 20009-4432
202-483-6622

State Hot Lines

Alabama
800-228-0469

Alaska
800-478-2437

Arizona
800-548-4695

Arkansas
800-342-2437

California (north)
800-367-2437

California (south)
800-400-7432

Colorado
800-252-2437

Connecticut
860-509-7801

Delaware
800-422-0429

District of Columbia
202-332-2437

Florida
800-243-7101

Georgia
800-551-2728

Hawaii
800-321-1555

Idaho
800-677-2437

Illinois
800-243-2437

Indiana
800-276-6443

Iowa
800-445-2437

Kansas
A hotline number is not available.

Kentucky
800-420-7431

Louisiana
800-922-4379

Maine
800-851-2437

Maryland
800-638-6252

Massachusetts
800-235-2331

Michigan
800-827-2437

Minnesota
800-248-2437

Mississippi
800-826-2961

Missouri
800-533-2437

Montana
800-233-6668

Nebraska
800-782-2437

Nevada
800-842-2437

New Hampshire
800-752-2437

New Jersey
800-624-2377

New Mexico
800-545-2437

New York
800-872-2777

North Carolina
800-342-2437

North Dakota
800-472-2180

Ohio
800-332-2437

Oklahoma
800-535-2437

Oregon
800-777-2437

Pennsylvania
800-662-6080

Puerto Rico
800-981-5721

Rhode Island
800-726-3010

South Carolina
800-322-2437

South Dakota
800-592-1861

Tennessee
800-525-2437

Texas
800-299-2437

Utah
800-366-2437

Vermont
800-882-2437

Virginia
800-533-4148

Virgin Islands
800-773-2437

Washington
800-272-2437

West Virginia
800-642-8244

Wisconsin
414-273-2437

Wyoming
800-327-3577

Internet Web Sites

Please note that web site addresses frequently change. The addresses provided here
were accurate at the time this section was prepared.

Advocates for Youth
http://www.advocatesforyouth.org

AIDS Clinical Trials Information Services (ACTIS)
http://www.actis.org

American Alliance for Health, Physical Education, Recreation and Dance
http://www.aahperd.org

American Journal of Nursing
http://www.ajn.org/journals/page1.cfm

American Journal of Public Health
http://www.apha.org/news/publications/journal/AJPH2.html

American Medical Association
http://www.ama-assn.org

American Medical News
http://www.ama-assn.org/public/journals/amnews/amnews.htm

Annals of Internal Medicine
http://www.acponline.org/journals/annals/annaltoc.htm

Ask NOAH About AIDS and HIV
http://www.noah.cuny.edu/aids/aids.html

Center for AIDS Prevention Studies at the University of California, San Francisco
http://www.caps.ucsf.edu

Centers for Disease Control and Prevention
http://www.cdc.gov

Food and Drug Administration
http://www.fda.gov

Healthfinder Information
http://www.healthfinder.org
(This government-sponsored site enables people to get reliable health information
faster and easier over the Internet.)

HIV/AIDS Surveillance Report
http://www.cdc.gov/nchstp/hiv_aids/stats/hasrlink.htm

HIV/AIDS Treatment Information Service
http://www.hivatis.org/atishome.html

HIV InfoWeb
http://www.infoweb.org

Journal of the American Medical Association
http://www.ama-assn.org/public/journals/jama/jamahome.htm

National Institutes of Health
http://www.nih.gov

National Library of Medicine
http://www.nlm.nih.gov
(This web site has Internet Grateful Med, which provides free access to MEDLINE, AIDSLINE, AIDSDRUGS, and AIDSTRIALS. The site also has PubMed, which provides free access to MEDLINE. These can be accessed through **http://www.nlm.nih.gov/databases/freemedl.html**)

Pan American Health Organization
http://www.oas.org/EN/PINFO/OAS/OLORGA4E.htm

The Lancet
http://www.thelancet.com

The New England Journal of Medicine
http://www.nejm.org

United Nations AIDS Programme
http://www.unaids.org

United Nations Children's Fund
http://www.unicef.org

World Health Organization
http://www.who.org

Index

About the Editors

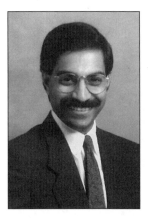

Gopal Sankaran, MD, DrPH, MNAMS, CHES, is a Professor of Public Health in the Department of Health at West Chester University of Pennsylvania. He is a physician, public health specialist, and health educator. He has a doctor of medicine (MD) degree from All India Institute of Medical Sciences and a master's and doctoral degrees in public health (MPH and DrPH) from the University of California at Berkeley. He is board certified in Integrated Maternal and Child Health Care and is an inducted member of the National Academy of Medical Sciences (MNAMS), India. He also is a Certified Health Education Specialist (CHES). He has worked as a consultant with the World Health Organization in Geneva in the Global Programme on AIDS and with PLAN International and Childreach on international HIV/AIDS prevention and control projects. He has received grants to research knowledge, attitudes, and practices of high school students, college students, and university faculty about HIV/AIDS. He has secured grants for HIV/AIDS prevention, published several articles in professional journals, and made numerous presentations on the topic at national, state, and local professional conferences.

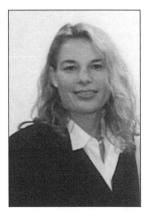

Karin A. E. Volkwein, PhD, is Associate Professor of Philosophy/History/Sociology of Sport and Physical Education in the Department of Kinesiology at West Chester University of Pennsylvania. During the summers, she is a standing visiting professor at the German Sport University in Cologne, Germany. Her research and teaching in the areas of sport philosophy, history, and sociology are based on an interdisciplinary approach with a cross-cultural comparative focus. Her research outcomes have been disseminated widely, both nationally and internationally, through numerous presentations, journal articles, and book chapters. She has served as guest editor for the *Social Science Review Special Issue on Sport Philosophy—1996* and is the editor of the forthcoming book *Fitness as a Cultural Phenomenon* (1997) from Waxmann Verlag. She has received numerous research grants and awards. One of her main research focuses is the topic HIV and sport. She also has served in various professional societies, such as the Philosophic Society of the Study of Sport (PSSS) and the Club of Cologne, and is currently chairing the Academy of Sport Philosophy under the American Alliance for Health, Physical

Education, Recreation and Dance (AAHPERD).

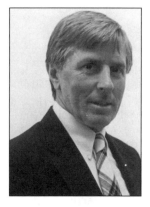

Dale R. Bonsall, MEd, is Associate Professor for Coaching and Pedagogy in the Department of Kinesiology at West Chester University of Pennsylvania. He has been involved with wrestling for over 30 years at the national and international levels, both as an athlete and a coach. He works with elite athletes of the U.S. Olympic Wrestling Team. He has conducted numerous clinics in wrestling over the years and has widely presented about issues related to wrestling. His expertise, practical engagement, and research interest about the topic HIV and sport has lead to several publications, both at the national and international levels.

List of Contributors

Jennifer M. Beller, PhD, is an Associate Professor at Eastern Michigan University and Affiliate Faculty Member at The Center for ETHICS at the University of Idaho.

Keith Gilbert, PhD, is currently on the Faculty of Health in the School of Human Movement Studies at Queensland University of Technology (QUT) at Brisbane, Australia.

Jack Harvey, MD, is the Chief Physician for USA Wrestling and a member of the Fédération Internationale des Luttes Associées (FILA) Medical Commission.

Mary A. Hums, MBA, MA, PhD, is an Associate Professor of Sport Administration at the University of Louisville, Kentucky.

Rodger L. Jackson, PhD, is an Assistant Professor at Richard Stockton College of New Jersey.

Deborah L. Keyser graduated from West Chester University and is currently teaching in Radnor School District in Pennsylvania.

Corrie J. Odom, DPT, MS, ATC, is currently a Physical Therapist at Kessler Memorial Hospital Rehabilitation Services in New Jersey.

Bente Klarlund Pedersen, MD, DrMedSci, is a senior registrar and leader of the immunologic laboratory of the Department of Infectious Diseases at the National University Hospital in Copenhagen, Denmark.

Sharon Kay Stoll, PhD. is Professor of Physical Education and the Director of The Center for ETHICS. She is a Distinguished Faculty Member and winner of a prestigious University Award for Teaching at the University of Idaho at Moscow.

Greg Strobel, MA, is the head coach of wrestling at Lehigh University in Pennsylvania. He is also the Chairman of the USA Wrestling Coaches Council.

Other books from Human Kinetics

Management of Bloodborne Infections in Sport

Terry A. Zeigler, MA
1997 • Paper • 96 pp • Item BZEI0682
ISBN 0-88011-682-X • $18.00 ($26.95 Cdn)

Shows sports personnel how to protect their athletes and themselves against serious bloodborne pathogens such as HIV and hepatitis B virus.

The Steroids Game

Charles Yesalis and Virginia Cowart
Foreword by Joe Paterno
1998 • Paper • 216 pp • Item PYES0494
ISBN 0-88011-494-0 • $16.95 ($24.95 Cdn)

Provides a straightforward and balanced discussion of what steroids are, how they work, their effects on athletic performance, and their health consequences.

Clinical Experiences in Athletic Training— A Modular Approach

Kenneth L. Knight, PhD, ATC
1998 • Spiral • 160 pp • Item BKNI0950
ISBN 0-87322-950-9 • $24.00 ($35.95 Cdn)

Second edition of Ken Knight's popular text features an improved, flexible approach to developing the appropriate clinical skills athletic trainers need.

The Clinical Orthopedic Assessment Guide

Janice Loudon, Stephania Bell, and Jane Johnston
1998 • Paper • 239 pp • Item BLOU0507
ISBN 0-88011-507-6 • $29.00 ($43.50 Cdn)

The only comprehensive, easy-to-use reference that includes all the vital information needed to perform orthopedic assessments.

Related Journal from Human Kinetics

Athletic Therapy Today

Frequency: Bimonthly (January, March, May, July, September, November)
Call for current subscription rates
ISSN: 1078-7895 • Item: JATT

To request more information or to order, U.S. customers call 1-800-747-4457, e-mail us at humank@hkusa.com or visit our Web site at www.humankinetics.com. Persons outside the U.S. can contact us via our Web site or use the appropriate telephone number, postal address, or e-mail address shown in the front of this book.

 HUMAN KINETICS
The Information Leader in Physical Activity